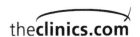

CLINICS IN GERIATRIC MEDICINE

Sleep in Elderly Adults

GUEST EDITOR
Julie K. Gammack, MD

February 2008 • Volume 24 • Number 1

SAUNDERS

An Imprint of Elsevier, Inc.
PHILADELPHIA   LONDON   TORONTO   MONTREAL   SYDNEY   TOKYO

W.B. SAUNDERS COMPANY
A Division of Elsevier Inc.

Elsevier, Inc. • 1600 John F. Kennedy Blvd., Suite 1800 • Philadelphia, PA 19103-2899

http://www.theclinics.com

CLINICS IN GERIATRIC MEDICINE
February 2008
Editor: Lisa Richman

Volume 24, Number 1
ISSN 0749-0690
ISBN-13: 978-1-4160-6050-5
ISBN-10: 1-4160-6050-2

The ideas and opinions expressed in the *Clinics in Geriatric Medicine* do not necessarily reflect those of the Publisher. The Publisher does not assume any responsibility for any injury and/or damage to persons or property arising out of or related to any use of the material contained in this periodical. The reader is advised to check the appropriate medical literature and the product information currently provided by the manufacturer of each drug to be administered to verify the dosage, the method and duration of administration, or contraindications. It is the responsibility of the treating physician or other health care professional, relying on independent experience and knowledge of the patient, to determine drug dosages and the best treatment for the patient. Mention of any product in this issue should not be construed as endorsement by the contributors, editors, or the Publisher of the product of manufacturers' claims.

Clinics in Geriatric Medicine (ISSN 0749-0690) is published quarterly by Elsevier Inc., 360 Park Avenue South, New York, NY 10010-1710. Months of issue are February, May, August, and November. Business and Editorial Offices: 1600 John F. Kennedy Blvd., Suite 1800, Philadelphia, PA 191023-2899. Customer Service Office: 6277 Sea Harbor Drive, Orlando, FL 32887-4800. Periodicals postage paid at New York, NY, and additional mailing offices. Subscription prices is $189.00 per year (US individuals), $327.00 per year (US institutions), $246.00 per year (Canadian individuals), $398.00 per year (Canadian institutions), $246.00 per year (foreign individuals) and $398.00 per year (foreign institutions). Foreign air speed delivery is included in all *Clinics* subscription prices. All prices are subject to change without notice. POSTMASTER: Send address changes to *Clinics in Geriatric Medicine*, Elsevier Periodicals Customer Service, 6277 Sea Harbor Drive, Orlando, FL 32887-4800. **Customer Service: 1-800-654-2452 (US). From outside of the US, call 1-407-345-4000.** E-mail: hhspcs@wbsaunder.com.

Clinics in Geriatric Medicine is covered in *Index Medicus, EMBASE/Excerpta Medica, Current Contents/ Clinical Medicine (CC/CM), and the Cumulative Index to Nursing & Allied Health Literature.*

Printed and bound by CPI Group (UK) Ltd, Croydon, CR0 4YY

Transferred to Digital Print 2011

GUEST EDITOR

JULIE K. GAMMACK, MD, Assistant Professor of Medicine, Division of Geriatric Medicine, Saint Louis University Health Sciences Center; GRECC, St. Louis VA Medical Center, St. Louis, Missouri

CONTRIBUTORS

SONIA ANCOLI-ISRAEL, PhD, Professor, Department of Psychiatry, University of California, San Diego, La Jolla, California; Department of Psychiatry, Veteran's Affairs San Diego Healthcare System, San Diego, California

JOSEPH ROLAND D. ESPIRITU, MD, FCCP, FAASM, Assistant Professor of Internal Medicine, Division of Pulmonary, Critical Care, and Sleep Medicine, Saint Louis University School of Medicine, St. Louis, Missouri

JOSEPH H. FLAHERTY, MD, Geriatric Research, Education and Clinical Center, St. Louis VA Medical Center; Associate Professor, Department of Internal Medicine, Division of Geriatrics, Saint Louis University School of Medicine, St. Louis, Missouri

JULIE K. GAMMACK, MD, Assistant Professor of Medicine, Division of Geriatric Medicine, Saint Louis University Health Sciences Center; GRECC, St. Louis VA Medical Center, St. Louis, Missouri

AIMÉE DINORAH GARCIA, MD, CWS, FCCWS, Assistant Professor, Department of Medicine, Geriatrics Section, Baylor College of Medicine, Houston, Texas

NALAKA S. GOONERATNE, MD, MSc, ABSM, Assistant Professor, Division of Geriatric Medicine, Center for Sleep and Respiratory Neurobiology; Associate Program Director, Clinical and Translational Science Award, University of Pennsylvania School of Medicine, Philadelphia, Pennsylvania

RAMZI R. HAJJAR, MD, Associate Professor of Medicine, Department of Internal Medicine, Division of Geriatric Medicine, St. Louis University School of Medicine; Geriatric Research, Education, and Clinical Center (GRECC), St. Louis Veterans' Affairs Medical Center, St. Louis, Missouri

MAGDOLNA HORNYAK, MD, Sleep Disorders Center, Department of Psychiatry and Psychotherapy, University Hospital Freiburg, Freiburg, Germany

SEEMA JOSHI, MD, Bettendorf Internal Medicine and Geriatrics, Bettendorf, Iowa

JOSÉ S. LOREDO, MD, MS, MPH, FCCP, Associate Professor of Clinical Medicine, Division of Pulmonary and Critical Care Medicine, University of California–San Diego School of Medicine, San Diego, California

BETH A. MALOW, MD, MS, Associate Professor, Department of Neurology, Vanderbilt University Medical Center; and Medical Director, Vanderbilt Sleep Disorders Center, Vanderbilt University Medical Center, Nashville, Tennessee

JENNIFER L. MARTIN, PhD, Research Health Scientist, Veteran's Affairs Greater Los Angeles Healthcare System, Geriatric Research, Education and Clinical Center, North Hills; and Assistant Research Professor, University of California, Los Angeles School of Medicine, Multicampus Program in Geriatric Medicine and Gerontology, Los Angeles, California

SUMI MISRA, MD, MPH, Assistant Professor of Medicine and Geriatrics, Division of General Internal Medicine, Vanderbilt University Medical Center, Nashville VA Hospital; and Director, Geriatrics Primary Care Clinics, Tennessee Valley Health Care System, Veterans Affairs Hospital, Nashville, Tennessee

DANIEL NORMAN, MD, Division of Pulmonary and Critical Care Medicine, University of California–San Diego School of Medicine, San Diego, California

MIGUEL A. PANIAGUA, MD, Assistant Professor of Medicine, Division of Gerontology & Geriatric Medicine, Saint Louis University School of Medicine, St. Louis, Missouri

ELIZABETH W. PANIAGUA, MD, St. Louis, Missouri

SHAILAJA PULISETTY, MD, Department of Internal Medicine, Division of Geriatrics, Saint Louis University School of Medicine, St. Louis, Missouri

KAI SPIEGELHALDER, Dipl.-Psych., Sleep Disorders Center, Department of Psychiatry and Psychotherapy, University Hospital Freiburg, Freiburg, Germany

SYED H. TARIQ, MD, FACP, Associate Professor of Internal Medicine and Geriatrics, Department of Internal Medicine, Division of Geriatrics, Saint Louis University School of Medicine, St. Louis, Missouri

CONTENTS

Obstructive Sleep Apnea in Older Adults

Daniel Norman and José S. Loredo

The "typical" presentation of obstructive sleep apnea (OSA) is chronic loud snoring and excessive daytime sleepiness in middle-aged obese men. OSA can result in increased risk for cardiovascular morbidity and mortality. The diagnostic features of OSA in older adults are similar to those in younger adults; however, the older adult may be less likely to seek medical attention or have the sleep disorder recognized because symptoms of snoring, sleepiness, fatigue, nocturia, unintentional napping, and cognitive dysfunction may be ascribed to the aging process itself or to other disorders. This article reviews the basic terminology and pathophysiology of sleep-disordered breathing, discusses why OSA may be even more prevalent in older adults than in the middle-aged group, and reviews similarities and differences between the two groups in the manifestations, consequences, and treatments of OSA.

Restless Legs Syndrome in Older Adults

Kai Spiegelhalder and Magdolna Hornyak

Restless legs syndrome (RLS) is a common neurological disorder characterized by an urge to move the legs. The symptoms show a strong circadian rhythmicity, with onset or increase in the evening or at night; thus, sleep disturbances are the most frequent reason for patients seeking medical aid. The prevalence of the disorder increases strongly with age, with an estimated 9% to 20% of sufferers being among the elderly. Dopaminergic drugs are the first-line treatment option in RLS; opioids and anticonvulsants can also be used either as add-on or stand alone therapy options. Secondary forms of RLS and possible interaction with other medications require particular consideration in the elderly.

FORTHCOMING ISSUES

May 2008

Pain Management
Howard Smith, MD, *Guest Editor*

August 2008

Diabetes
John Morley, MD, *Guest Editor*

PREVIOUS ISSUES

November 2007

Gastroenterology
Syed Tariq, MD, FACP, *Guest Editor*

May 2007

Emergencies in the Elderly Patient
Amal Mattu, MD, Michael Winters, MD,
and Katherine Grundmann, MD, *Guest Editors*

February 2007

Heart Failure in the Elderly
Wilbert S. Aronow, MD, *Guest Editor*

THE CLINICS ARE NOW AVAILABLE ONLINE!

Access your subscription at:
www.theclinics.com

ELSEVIER
SAUNDERS

Clin Geriatr Med 24 (2008) xi–xiii

CLINICS IN
GERIATRIC
MEDICINE

Preface

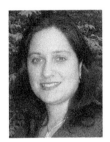

Julie K. Gammack, MD
Guest Editor

Many things—such as loving, going to sleep, or behaving unaffectedly—are done worst when we try hardest to do them.

—*C.S. Lewis (British Scholar and Novelist, 1898–1963)*

The need to sleep and obtain adequate rest is an essential bodily function from birth to death. Like eating and breathing, sleep is necessary for human survival. Sleep patterns evolve as one moves from infancy to childhood and into adulthood. It should be no surprise, then, that sleep parameters also evolve as the body enters the oldest decades of life.

Insomnia is a subjective report of insufficient or nonrestorative sleep despite the opportunity to get adequate rest. A person's perception of "inadequate sleep" may in fact be erroneously affected by culture, societal norms, and misinformation about aging. In the United States, the prevalence of sleep disturbances ranges from 30%–60% [1,2]. As with many symptoms attributed to "just getting old," one must be cautious about assuming that poor sleep is an aging-related phenomenon.

Many sleep parameters do change with aging, but should not inherently result in fatigue or disrupted daytime functioning. It is necessary for clinicians to understand the physiology of sleep in older adults and the differences between expected aging and disease. This information can then be used to educate patients and their families on typical sleep patterns of older adults. Establishing appropriate sleep expectations and correcting misperceptions can alleviate sleep anxiety and reduced dissatisfaction with insomnia management.

0749-0690/08/$ - see front matter © 2008 Elsevier Inc. All rights reserved.
doi:10.1016/j.cger.2007.08.014   *geriatric.theclinics.com*

Aging-related changes in any body system are influenced by genetically predetermined physiology, environmental stressors, and accumulated disease states. The need for sleep, like other bodily functions, is affected throughout the lifespan by these forces. Primary sleep disturbances such as sleep apnea and restless legs syndrome are seen with increasing frequency in the elderly. Comorbid diseases also increase with age and can impact sleep primarily or secondarily. Dementing illnesses and certain medications alter the normal neurohormonal balance, disrupting the circadian cycle of sleep. Other illnesses and medications may contribute to pain, dyspnea, or other symptoms that subsequently preclude restful sleep.

Conversely, inadequate or dysfunctional sleep results in a multitude of physical, functional, and cognitive impairments in both quality of life and longevity. An increased rate of falls, cognitive decline, and even death has been associated with poor sleep in older adults [3–5]. Discerning those conditions that contribute to, and those that result from, poor sleep may be challenging. Cause and effect may be intertwined, not unlike many complex conditions of the elderly.

Causes of poor sleep may be intrinsic, involving disease and medications, or extrinsic, of environmental or behavioral origin. Perhaps it would be better to designate insomnia in the older adult as one of many geriatric syndromes to conditions of multifactorial etiology requiring a multidimensional approach to diagnosis and management. Without identifying all possible contributions to poor sleep, and instituting a multifaceted management strategy, successful treatment for insomnia may be elusive.

Nonpharmacologic interventions such as cognitive-behavioral therapy (CBT), alteration in sleep environment, and treatment of sleep-disrupting disease symptoms can be quite effective in managing sleep disturbances. With proper education and a motivated participant, improvement in sleep with these techniques can be attained with older adults. Morin and colleagues conducted a randomized-controlled trial of CBT versus conventional pharmacologic treatment for primary insomnia in 78 adults (mean age = 65). A 55% reduction in nocturnal awake time was seen with CBT compared with a 47% reduction in the medication group. Sustained sleep improvement was greater in the CBT group [6]. A meta-analysis of both pharmacologic and nonpharmacologic treatments for insomnia also demonstrated short-term sleep benefits with CBT similar to those seen with pharmacologic treatment [7].

For many conditions, including insomnia, pharmacologic treatment is an effective and efficient means of alleviating disease symptoms. Many classes of prescription and nonprescription drugs alter the sleep cycle and induce a more satisfactory sleep quality. A recent meta-analysis demonstrated that sedative-hypnotic medications are effective in improving sleep quality in older adults with an odds ratio of 0.14 (95% CI, 0.05–0.23) compared with placebo [8].

However, like most pharmacotherapies in older adults, side effects are more prevalent and potentially more dangerous. The intended sleep side effects of fatigue and drowsiness are also risk factors for confusion and dizziness in older adults. In this same study, adverse cognitive events with sedative-hypnotic use were reported with an odds ratio of 4.78 (95% CI, 1.47–15.47). The mantra "start low, go slow" is even more true when using sleep-inducing medications in older adults.

For the clinician, managing insomnia requires understanding aging-related sleep physiology, conditions resulting from poor sleep, and diseases (primary and secondary) that are detrimental to sleep quality. Managing the comorbidities that contribute to poor sleep is necessary but may not be sufficient in treating insomnia in older adults. Finding a balance between pharmacologic and nonpharmacologic strategies is part of a multi-dimensional treatment plan for older adults. When pharmacologic intervention is indicated, balancing the potential side effects with realistic benefits can lead to a more satisfactory and sustained result for the patient.

In this issue of *Clinics in Geriatric Medicine*, "Sleep Disorders in Older Adults," the spectrum of sleep-related changes and disease states is discussed. Evaluation of insomnia is summarized in the context of the elderly individual. Sleep disturbances are specifically reviewed in various care settings and disease states. Finally, this issue discusses both pharmacologic and nonpharmacologic management of sleep disorders to provide a multidimensional array of treatment options for the medical provider.

Julie K. Gammack, MD
Saint Louis University Health Sciences Center (GRECC)
St. Louis VA Medical Center
St. Louis, MO 63125-4199, USA

References

[1] Schubert CR, Cruickshanks KJ, Dalton DS, et al. Prevalence of sleep problems and quality of life in an older population. Sleep 2002;25:889–93.
[2] Foley DJ, Monjan AA, Brown SL, et al. Sleep complaints among elderly persons: an epidemiologic study of three communities. Sleep 1995;18:425–32.
[3] Brassington GS, King AC, Bliwise DL. Sleep problems as a risk factor for falls in a sample of community-dwelling adults aged 64–99 years. J Am Geriatr Soc 2000;48:1234–40.
[4] Cricco M, Simonsick EM, Foley DJ. The impact of insomnia on cognitive functioning in older adults. J Am Geriatr Soc 2001;29:1184–9.
[5] Manabe K, Matsui T, Yamaya M, et al. Sleep patterns and mortality among elderly patients in a geriatric hospital. Gerontology 2000;46:318–22.
[6] Morin CM, Colecchi C, Stone J, et al. Behavioral and pharmacological therapies for late-life insomnia. A randomized controlled trial. JAMA 1999;281:991–9.
[7] Smith MT, Perlis ML, Park A, et al. Comparative meta-analysis of pharmacotherapy and behavior therapy for persistent insomnia. Am J Psychiatry 2002;150:5–11.
[8] Glass J, Lanctot KL, Hermann N, et al. Sedative hypnotics in older people with insomnia: meta-analysis of risks and benefits. BMJ 2005;331:1169.

ELSEVIER
SAUNDERS

CLINICS IN
GERIATRIC
MEDICINE

Clin Geriatr Med 24 (2008) 1–14

Aging-Related Sleep Changes

Joseph Roland D. Espiritu, MD, FCCP, FAASM

*Division of Pulmonary, Critical Care, and Sleep Medicine, Saint Louis University School
of Medicine, 3635 Vista Avenue at Grand Boulevard, PO Box 15250, Saint Louis,
MO 63110-0250, USA*

Normal aging results in changes in the function of all organ systems and impacts the neurophysiology of sleep. Most physicians who care for the elderly may have the general impression that aging results in the deterioration in the quality of sleep and an increase in the prevalence of sleep disorders. This impression was validated by a large epidemiological study of over 9,000 elderly subjects in three United States communities in 1995, which described that the vast majority (more than 80%) of them had one or more sleep complaints, such as trouble falling asleep, waking up, awaking too early, needing to nap, and not feeling rested [1]. On the other hand, in a study of another, much older, population, good quality sleep was surprisingly reported by the majority of this cohort. An analysis of the presence of sleep disorders, their related pathologies, and pharmacologic treatments in 180 Roman centenarians revealed that more than half (57.4%) had good quality sleep [2]. In general, predictors of good quality sleep in the elderly include physical and psychologic health, daytime activity, and naturalistic light (3000+ lux) [3]. On the other hand, moderate impairment in sleep quality in these Roman centenarians was found in about one third (35.2%) and was associated with cardiopulmonary comorbidities (angina pectoris and chronic obstructive pulmonary disease). A small minority (7.4%) manifested severe impairments in sleep quality significantly associated with cognitive dysfunction and increased mortality [2]. Thus, an increase in the number of sleep complaints may be a marker of poor physical and mental health [4].

This article describes the normal changes in sleep physiology in the elderly. Distinguishing "normal" or physiologic age-related changes in sleep from "abnormal" or pathologic sleep can be problematic, given the close association between sleep disorders and a higher prevalence of comorbid conditions in the elderly. In an attempt to ensure that the age-related changes

---

E-mail address: espiritu@slu.edu

0749-0690/08/$ - see front matter © 2008 Elsevier Inc. All rights reserved.
doi:10.1016/j.cger.2007.08.007
geriatric.theclinics.com

described herein are indeed physiologic and not associated with adverse health effects, this article focuses mainly on studies that incorporate healthy elderly subjects and compares them to younger adults as controls. Specific sleep disorders that increase in prevalence with aging (sleep breathing disorders, insomnia, restless legs syndrome, rapid eye movement behavior disorder, and so on) are discussed elsewhere in this issue.

Sleep initiation and maintenance

Several reports suggest that the ability to initiate and maintain sleep declines with aging. Sleep in older adults tend to become shorter (decreased total sleep time), more shallow (increased stages 1 and 2 and decreased slow-wave sleep), and more disrupted (decreased sleep efficiency, increased arousal index, and prolonged wake after sleep onset) [4–7]. Mathematical modeling reveals that the rate of increase in initial sleep latency over the ages is not linear but triphasic, increasing until age 30, plateauing between ages 30 and 50, and then resuming its upward climb after age 50 [8]. Sleep efficiency continues to deteriorate in the old elderly (over 70 years old), with an additional increase in the wake time (plus 28 minutes per decade of life), at the expense of stages 1 and 2 (minus 24 minutes per decade) and stage rapid eye movement (REM) sleep (minus 10 minutes per decade) [6]. A meta-analysis published by Floyd and colleagues [9] on age-related changes in the initiation and maintenance of sleep confirmed that waking frequency (arousal index) and duration (wake after sleep onset) increased with aging. However, older subjects appear to be somewhat less cognizant of this impaired ability to initiate and maintain sleep. They tend to underestimate the severity of sleep impairment (ie, longer sleep latency, less total sleep time, lower sleep time) when their self-report is tested against polysomnography [3,10]. Meanwhile, although healthy older people have a greater number of arousals during their nocturnal sleep period, their ability to reinitiate sleep remains surprisingly intact and comparable to those of younger individuals [11].

The decreased ability to initiate and maintain sleep is unfortunately associated with increased morbidity and mortality in the elderly. A prolonged sleep latency at or above the 95th percentile (greater than or equal to 80 minutes) in a cohort of older Parisians (over 60 years old) was associated with anxiety, poor health, insomnia, and obstructive sleep apnea [12]. In a prospective study by Dew and colleagues [13] of 185 healthy older adults 60 to 89 years old, and with no history of neurocognitive deficits, predictors of all-cause mortality (controlled for age, sex, gender, and baseline medical burden) include a prolonged initial sleep latency (more than 30 minutes), poor sleep efficiency (less than 80%), and increased (over 25.7%) or decreased (less than 16.1%) proportion of REM sleep.

Sleep duration

A number of elderly patients complain about not getting enough sleep. Although this perception of decreased sleep duration may be attributable to the circadian phase advancement of the sleep-wake schedule in the elderly (ie, waking up early in the morning while the rest of the household members are asleep), or the effect of shortened nocturnal sleep because of daytime napping, measuring the actual time spent sleeping during the 24-hour period, using subjective and objective tools, is key to ascertaining this phenomenon. Campbell and Murphy [14], compared spontaneous sleep among young, middle-age, and older adults, using the disentrainment protocol, where subjects slept for 72 hours while being shielded from natural and artificial cues to time of day, with the goal of determining the duration of spontaneous sleep. Total sleep time over 24 hours was significantly shorter in the middle-age (9.06 hours) and older age (8.13 hours) adults than that in the younger ones (10.53 hours).

Sleep duration appears to be a predictor of an older individual's state of health and longevity. In the Japanese Collaborative Cohort Study on Evaluation of Cancer Risk involving 104,010 subjects aged 40 to 79 years, the optimal sleep duration associated with the lowest risk mortality was found to be 7 hours [15]. Longer or shorter sleep times were associated with increased all-cause mortality. In a study of a Mediterranean population that practiced siesta, men who slept more than 8 hours per day (versus those who slept less than 8 hours per day) had double the risk of dying from all causes and almost triple the risk from heart disease [16]. Furthermore, short and long nocturnal sleep duration may also indicate the presence of comorbid conditions in the elderly. Ohayon and Vecchierini [12] studied the relationship between sleep duration and cognitive function in older adults in 7,010 randomly selected metropolitan Parisian households, and found that extremes in sleep duration may indicate the presence of health risk factors. Those older individuals with nocturnal sleep durations at or below the 5th percentile (4 hours and 30 minutes) had a significantly higher prevalence of obesity, poor health, insomnia, daytime sleepiness, and cognitive impairment. At the other extreme, those total nocturnal sleep times at or above the 95th percentile (9 hours and 30 minutes) were more likely to be male, anxious, less educated, unhealthy, insomniac, or apneic.

Sleep schedule

The current available literature supports the widely held belief that the nocturnal sleep phase is shifted earlier in the elderly. In an interesting study of Japanese office workers divided into four age groups (20s, 30s, 40s, and 50s–60s) using a morningness-eveningness questionnaire, Ishihara and colleagues [17] not only reaffirmed that older workers preferred earlier bed and arising times, but also observed that they had a less variable sleep schedule and better mood upon arising, compared with younger workers. This preference for earlier bedtimes was further supported by another study, which demonstrated that later bedtimes are associated not only with less time in bed but also less time asleep. For each 10 minute-delay in bedtime starting after 19:00 hours, there was a corresponding 7 to 8 minute decrement in time in bed and total sleep time [18]. Extremes in bedtime or wake-up time may also indicate an older person's state of health. The Ohayon's study on older Parisians concluded that early (9 PM or earlier) or late (1 AM or later) bedtime, as well as extremely early (5 AM or earlier) and later (9 AM or later) wake-up times were associated with obesity and loss of autonomy in the activities of daily living [12].

Naps

A polysomnographic study, incorporating young adults (20–30 years old) as controls, found a greater number of naps in older adults (over 78 years old) [19]. An uncontrolled, observational study employing an activity diary and wrist actigraphy found that healthy elderly individuals spent approximately one hour napping during the day [20]. In the general population, daytime napping may have salutary effects on health outcomes. In the Greek European Prospective Investigation Into Cancer and Nutrition study of 23,681 healthy individuals, siesta was associated with a 37% lower coronary mortality, especially in working men [21].

There are a few studies published investigating the effect of naps on polysomnographic parameters and neurocognitive function in the healthy elderly population. Monk and colleagues [22] performed a 17-day, 90-minute nap versus no nap interventional study on nine healthy elderly subjects aged 74 to 87 years, and found a significant increment in total sleep time (38 minutes) and improvement in sleep latency (15.6 minutes versus 11.5 minutes, respectively) in a single-trial evening mutiple sleep latency test. Although nocturnal sleep efficiency dropped by a small proportion (2.4%) mainly because of earlier wake times, there were no reliable effects on wake after sleep onset or measures of non-REM (NREM) (stages 1, 2, and delta) sleep. On the other hand, Campbell and colleagues [23] performed polysomnography, body core temperature measurements, and neurocognitive testing on 32 healthy individuals aged 55 to 85 years and found that napping had little effect on subsequent nighttime sleep quality or duration, thereby significantly increasing their total 24-hour sleep time. These increased sleep times were associated with enhanced cognitive and psychomotor performance measured the following day.

Sleep architecture

The meta-analysis on age-related sleep changes, published by Ohayon and colleagues, [24] described the evolution of sleep architecture in healthy individuals from childhood to old age. Table 1 summarizes the age-related changes in sleep architecture based on current literature. The proportion of time spent in the shallower NREM sleep stages 1 and 2 increases with aging, mainly as a consequence of the decrease in proportion the more restorative slow-wave (stages 3 and 4, or N3) sleep. The mean percentage of slow-wave sleep decreases from 18.9% during early adulthood (16–25 years old) to 3.4% during midlife (36–50 years old) [25]. The largest decrease in delta sleep appears to occur during the first 100 minutes of sleep (NREM period 1) and during early adulthood (between 20 and 40 years old) [7]. There appears to be no further decrease in slow-wave sleep after age 70 years. Possible mechanisms for the decrease in slow-wave sleep in older individuals include the parallel decline in the growth hormone secretion [5] and the predominant loss of parasympathetic activity, as suggested by the decreased heart rate variability found in the elderly [26].

The same meta-analysis by Ohayon's group concluded that the proportion of REM sleep declined with aging [24]. The major decrement in REM sleep occurs between young and middle adulthood, after which no further change is noted. Meanwhile, the investigators also found a decrease in REM latency with age, a finding that may easily be confounded by concomitant psychiatric disorders, drugs, alcohol, and sleep disorders. In addition, the distribution of REM sleep throughout the night appears to shift the occurrence of REM sleep toward the earlier part on the night. REM sleep was increased in the first quarter of the sleep episode and the increment of REM sleep during the course of nocturnal sleep was diminished in the older age group [27]. Wauquier and colleagues [28] monitored the sleep-wake activity in 14 elderly individuals over the age of 88 using ambulatory polysomnography, and also found a shift of REM sleep toward the first part of the sleep period. Meanwhile, the stage from which sleep termination occurs appears to shift with aging. Murphy and colleagues [29] examined sleep termination in young adults (19–28 years old) and older adults (60–82 years old) and found that while younger ones arose preferentially from stage REM, older subjects were most likely to arise from a NREM sleep stage. In addition, older subjects with higher sleep efficiencies were more likely to also arise from stage REM.

Table 1
Age-related changes in polysomnographic characteristics

Increase	Decrease
Sleep latency	Total sleep time
Stage 1 sleep %	Sleep Efficiency
Stage 2 sleep %	Slow wave sleep %
Wake after sleep onset	REM sleep %
	REM latency

Sleep electrophysiology

Spectral analysis

Aging is associated with a reduction of power in the sleep EEG, as well as frequency-specific changes in the brain topography. Landolt and Borbely [5] performed spectral analysis of sleep EEG records comparing middle aged healthy men (mean age of 62 years) and young men (mean age of 22.3 years), and found that the age-related reduction of EEG power in NREM sleep (0.25 Hz–14 Hz) and REM sleep (0.75 Hz) is most pronounced in the anterior derivation (frontocentral) toward the middle (central-parietal) EEG derivation.

Sleep spindle and K-complex

The hallmarks of stage 2 sleep (sleep spindles and K complexes, [Fig. 1]) are also altered with aging. Crowley and colleagues [30] analyzed the properties of sleep spindles and K-complexes in 20 neurologically and medically healthy, older adults (mean age of 75.5 years) not taking psychoactive medications, and found a decrease in spindle number, density, and duration, as well as decrease in the number and density of K-complexes from young adult control values. They also found a subtle yet significant increase (plus 0.5 Hz) in the EEG frequency of spindles in the elderly. Nicolas and colleagues [31] corroborated the progressive decrease in sleep spindle number, density, and duration, as well as the progressive increase in intraspindle frequency with age. There also appears to be an altered circadian modulation of spindle frequency in older adults. In young adults, spindle density and amplitude are higher, while spindle frequency and its variability are lower during the biologic night (when melatonin secretion is high) than during the day. In contrast,

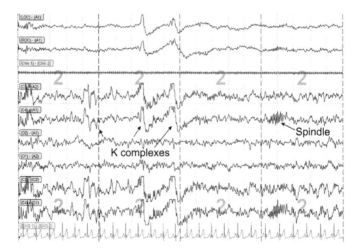

Fig. 1. Hallmarks of Stage N2 sleep: K complexes and spindles.

Knoblauch and colleagues [32], using a 40-hour multiple-nap design under constant-routine condition, detected a weaker circadian modulation (ie, decreased night-day difference and variability) of spindle frequency in older adults (57–74 years old). These changes in the generation of spindles and K-complexes may signify certain age-related changes in the thalamocortical regulatory mechanisms involving NREM sleep.

Delta activity

Aging not only decreases the time spent in slow-wave (stages 3 and 4 or stage N3) sleep, but also alters delta activity (Fig. 2). Smith and colleagues [33] analyzed all slow waves (greater than 5 muV in magnitude between 0.5 Hz and 3.0 Hz) during the first 6 hours of nocturnal sleep in 25 healthy subjects between 3 and 79 years old, and found that increasing age was associated with a decrement in the average peak amplitude of the delta waves, slowing of delta frequencies, and a decrease in the incidence of waves greater than 20 muV, particularly in the frontal areas. Meanwhile, Ehlers and Kupfer [7] evaluated sleep EEG's in 24 men without medical and psychiatric illness, classified them into three age groups (21–30, 31–40, and 51–70 years old) and performed computer-assisted delta and REM quantification, and power spectral analysis. While Ehlers group corroborated Smith's findings on the expected age-related decrease in delta activity, the former group found a shift in the spectral distribution of delta power toward the higher rather than lower frequencies.

Rapid eye movements

Aside from the decrease in REM sleep proportion and distribution during nocturnal sleep, REM density may be affected by aging. Darchia and colleagues [34] compared the eye movement density between elderly subjects and young adults who underwent EEG and extraoculography for four

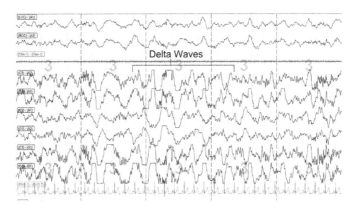

Fig. 2. Hallmark of Stage N3 (slow-wave sleep or Stages 3 and 4 sleep: delta waves).

nonconsecutive baseline nights, and found that the former had a significantly lower incidence of rapid eye movements. Further studies are needed to determine the neurocognitive implications of this decrease in REM activity in the elderly. In summary, aging is associated with changes in the electroencephalographic hallmarks of both NREM and REM sleep stages (Table 2).

Body movements during sleep

In a study comparing 12 elderly with 7 young healthy subjects, Gori and colleagues [35] found a significant general decrease in the number of body movements during sleep, from infancy to adulthood and even into the later ages. While body movements occurred predominantly during stage REM (ie, phasic twitching of the skeletal muscles) in the young adult, they were not specifically associated with any sleep state or stage in the elderly. The investigators attributed the loss of preferential occurrence of body movements during stage REM to the age-related change in the control of the subcortical circuits by the motor cortex. Moreover, body movements in the elderly appear to be significantly more disruptive of sleep than in the young adults, as they are more often followed by either a shift in the sleep state or a behavioral awakening.

Circadian rhythm

There is growing evidence that alteration of circadian rhythm (biologic sleep-wake clock) may partly be responsible for age-related sleep changes.

Table 2
Age-related changes in properties of sleep stage hallmarks

Sleep stage	Change in sleep stage hallmarks
Stage 2 (N2)	Decrease in spindle number
	Decrease in spindle density
	Decrease in spindle duration
	Increase in intraspindle frequency
	Attenuation in modulation (ie, decrease in night-day difference and variability) of spindle frequency by the circadian rhythm
	Decrease in the number of K complexes
	Decrease in the density of K complexes
Stages 3 and 4 (N3 or slow-wave sleep)	Decrease in the peak amplitude
	Decrease in the incidence of slow waves > 20 muV, especially in the frontal areas
Stage REM	Decrease in the incidence of rapid eye movements

Monk and colleagues [36] compared a group of 45 healthy older men and women (71–91 years old) with 21 young controls (19–28 years old) and found that despite the older group's similar social activities, involvement, and greater regularity in daily lifestyle than the younger group, the older group still had worse subjective and objective sleep as measured by the Pittsburgh Sleep Quality Index and nocturnal polysomnography, respectively. Because sleep disruption in the elderly cannot be blamed solely upon the age-related changes in daily social activities, it is, therefore, worthwhile to explore other possible mechanisms for these sleep changes in the elderly.

Several studies have detected alterations in the circadian modulation of sleep that may help explain findings, such as excessive daytime sleepiness, impaired sleep initiation and maintenance, altered sleep architecture, and phase-advanced sleep schedule in elderly individuals. Münch and colleagues [37] studied the circadian rhythms and spectral components of the sleep EEG in 17 young (20–31 year old) and 15 older (57–74 year old) volunteers under constant posture conditions during a 40-hour nap protocol (75-minute sleep and 150-minute wake schedule). The investigators concluded that aging is associated with a weaker circadian arousal signal, based on the increased occurrence of sleep episodes during the wake maintenance zone and the higher subjective sleepiness ratings in the late afternoon and evening in the older group. They also found a diminished melatonin secretion and a reduced circadian modulation of REM sleep, together with less pronounced day-night differences in the lower alpha and spindle range of sleep EEG activity in the older group.

Cajochen and colleagues [38] compared the responses of a group of healthy older volunteers with those of younger adults to sleep deprivation protocol (high sleep pressure condition) versus a nap protocol (low sleep pressure condition). They also noted an age-related weakening of the circadian arousal signal based on the higher propensity for sleep during the wake maintenance zone, higher subjective sleepiness ratings in the late afternoon and evening, diminished melatonin secretion, and reduced circadian regulation of REM sleep and spindle frequency in the older subjects. Dijk and colleagues [27] investigated the circadian and homeostatic regulation of human sleep during forced desynchrony in 13 older men and women and 11 young men, and found that older people had reduced sleep duration at all circadian phases and that sleep consolidation deteriorated more rapidly during the course of sleep, especially when the second half of the sleep occurred after the crest of the melatonin rhythm.

Vitiello and colleagues [39] also noted age-related changes in the circadian temperature rhythms. Older men had higher temperatures at the nadir of the temperature curve and lower peak-to-trough temperature curve amplitudes than younger men. Czeisler and colleagues [40] corroborated this decreased amplitude of the endogenous circadian temperature oscillation, but also noted that its phase occurred almost 2 hours earlier in the older age group. Finally, in a study of 44 older subjects under a constant routine protocol, Duffy and colleagues [41] noted that although the average wake time and endogenous circadian phase of the older subjects did occur earlier than that of 101 young men, the older subjects' endogenous circadian temperature nadir occurred later than relative to their wake time when compared with the younger subjects. All of these studies demonstrate alterations in the circadian modulation of sleep that may be partly responsible for age-related changes in sleep quantity, quality, architecture, and schedule in the elderly.

Sleep deprivation

The deleterious neurocognitive effect of sleep deprivation in healthy older adults seems to be blunted. Bonnett [42] designed an experiment disrupting sleep 14 times per hour, using auditory stimulus, in 12 normal 55- to 70-year-old adults and another 12 normal young adults, and demonstrated that older subjects had a smaller increase in total awakenings during the second night of sleep disturbance and a slower increase in auditory arousal threshold as the sleep disturbance progressed. More interestingly, the older subjects had less performance deterioration in completing addition problems in the morning, when compared with the younger ones [18]. Adam and colleagues [43] compared the psychomotor vigilance task performance of 11 older men (mean age of 66.4 years) with a dozen healthy young men (mean age of 25.2 years) after 40 hours of prolonged wakefulness, and found that vigilant attention is less impaired in older men. In terms of age-related changes of the EEG responses to sleep deprivation, Münch and colleagues [44] subjected healthy young (20–31 year old) and older (57–74 year old) subjects to a 40-hour sleep deprivation protocol, and noted that the frontal predominance of delta activity after sleep loss decreased with aging.

Respiratory function during sleep

Age-related degenerative changes in respiratory function have been reported and may be partly responsible for the increased cardiovascular morbidity and mortality in the elderly. Naifeh and colleagues [45] compared the several respiratory variables in 11 healthy elderly subjects (older than 60 years) with 12 younger controls (30–39 years), and reported that the occurrence of sleep apneas, hypopneas, and arousals because of respiratory events were increased in the older subjects. Although there were transient swings in the pulse oximetry oxygen saturation and end-tidal and transcutaneous carbon dioxide tension associated with the respiratory events in the older subjects, their mean values were maintained during sleep at the expense of the loss of the sleep-related, physiologic drop in minute ventilation and tidal volume found in the younger subjects [44]. Meanwhile, Hudgel and colleagues [46] documented an increased prevalence of periodic breathing in healthy elderly individuals, which may be related to wide oscillations in upper airway resistance producing fluctuating hypoventilation. Degenerative changes in the hypercapnic ventilatory drive cannot be blamed for these changes in respiratory parameters. Browne and colleagues [47] compared the change in the hypercapnic ventilatory response from wakefulness to sleep between 10 elderly and 10 young individuals without sleep apnea, and found no difference. Further studies are needed to help elucidate the mechanisms underlying these age-related changes in respiratory function.

Endocrine function during sleep

The widely known age-related changes in neuroendocrine function have been responsible for the deterioration of health and quality of life in the elderly. Alterations in hormonal secretion during sleep may also be related to the impaired sleep quality in older adults. Sherman and colleagues [48] studied the effect of age on the circadian rhythm of plasma cortisol in 34 normal subjects, and demonstrated a negative correlation between age and the maximum cortisol secretion, the time of the nadir of the cortisol concentration, and the acrophase. Kern and colleagues [49] measured the changes in cortisol and growth hormone secretion during nocturnal sleep in 30 male volunteers, aged 20 to 92 years, and found that growth hormone secretion decreased while the cortisol nadir increased linearly as a function of age. Several studies have tried to correlate these age-related changes in cortisol and growth hormone secretion with sleep impairment in the elderly. Prinz and colleagues [50] measured the 24 hour urine-free cortisol levels in 88 healthy, older, nonobese men and women (mean age of 70.6 years) and observed that subjects with higher cortisol levels had more impaired sleep (lower sleep efficiency, fewer minutes of stages 2, 3, and 4 sleep, and more EEG beta activity during NREM sleep). Van Cauter and colleagues [25] noted a biphasic decline in growth hormone secretion: early adulthood to midlife is accompanied by a major decline in growth hormone secretion (minus 372 micrograms per decade) followed by a slower decline (minus 43 micrograms per decade) from mid- to late-life. This biphasic decline in growth hormone secretion correlated with a parallel decline in slow-wave sleep. They also detected an age threshold of 50 years of age, after which evening cortisol levels rose (plus 19.3 nmol/L per decade) together with worsening sleep fragmentation and decline in REM sleep. The above reported changes in nocturnal growth hormone and cortisol levels correlated significantly with an age-dependent decrease in slow-wave sleep and REM sleep, and may be partially responsible for the reduced restorative neurocognitive and anabolic functions of sleep in the aged.

Summary

Normal aging is accompanied by changes in the sleep quality, quantity, and architecture. Specifically, there appears to be a measurable decrease in the ability to initiate and maintain sleep accompanied by a decrease in the proportion of the deeper, more restorative slow-wave sleep and REM sleep in the healthy elderly. There is epidemiologic evidence that this impaired ability to initiate and maintain adequate sleep may be a marker of increased mortality and neurocognitive dysfunction. On the other hand, napping appears to have a salutary effect on neurocognitive function in the elderly. Possible mechanisms related to these age-related changes in sleep include age-related changes in circadian modulation, homeostatic factors, cardio-pulmonary function, and endocrine function.

References

[1] Foley DJ, Monjan AA, Brown SL, et al. Sleep complaints among elderly persons: an epide-miologic study of three communities. Sleep 1995;18:425–32.
[2] Tafaro L, Cicconetti P, Baratta A, et al. Sleep quality of centenarians: cognitive and survival implications. Arch Gerontol Geriatr 2007;44S:385–9.
[3] Hood B, Bruck D, Kennedy G. Determinants of sleep quality in the healthy aged: the role of physical, psychological, circadian, and naturalistic light variables. Age and Ageing 2004;33: 159–65.
[4] Reid KJ, Martinovich Z, Finkel S, et al. Sleep: a marker of physical and mental health in the elderly. Am J Geriatr Psychiatry 2006;14:860–8.
[5] Landolt HP, Borbely AA. Age-dependent changes in sleep EEG topography. Clin Neuro-physiol 2001;112:369–77.
[6] Webb WB. Sleep in older persons: sleeps structures of 50- to 60-year-old men and women. J Gerontol 1982;37:581–6.
[7] Ehlers CL, Kupfer DJ. Effects of age on delta and REM sleep parameters. Electroencepha-logr Clin Neurophysiol 1989;72:118–25.
[8] Floyd JA, Janisse JJ, Marshall MS, et al. Nonlinear components of age-related change in sleep initiation. Nurs Res 2000;49:290–4.
[9] Floyd JA, Medler SM, Ager JW, et al. Age-related changes in initiation and maintenance of sleep: a meta-analysis. Res Nurs Health 2000;23:106–17.
[10] Vitiello MV, Larsen LH, Moe KE. Age-related change: gender and estrogen effects on sub-jective-objective sleep quality relationships of healthy noncomplaining older men and women. J Psychosom Res 2004;56:503–10.
[11] Klerman EB, Davis JB, Duffy JF, et al. Older people awaken more frequently but fall back asleep at the same rate as younger people. Sleep 2004;27:793–8.
[12] Ohayon MM, Vecchierini MF. Normative sleep data, cognitive function, and daily living activities in older adults in the community. Sleep 2005;28:981–9.
[13] Dew MA, Hoch CC, Buysse DJ, et al. Healthy older adults' sleep predicts all-cause mortality at 4–19 years of follow-up. Psychosom Med 2003;65:63–73.
[14] Campbell S, Murphy P. The nature of spontaneous sleep across adulthood. J Sleep Res 2007; 16:24–32.
[15] Tamakoshi A, Ohno Y, JACC Study Group. Self-reported sleep duration as a predictor of all-cause mortality. Sleep 2004;27:51–4.
[16] Burazeri G, Gofin J, Kark JD. Over 8 hours of sleep—marker of increased mortality in Med-iterranean population: follow-up population study. Croat Med J 2003;44:193–8.
[17] Ishihara K, Miyake S, Miyasita A, et al. Morningness-eveningness preference and sleep habits in Japanese office workers of different ages. Chronobiologia 1992;19:9–16.
[18] Monk TH, Thompson WK, Buysse DJ, et al. Sleep in healthy seniors: a diary study of the relation between bedtime and the amount of sleep obtained. J Sleep Res 2006;15:256–60.

[19] Buysse DJ, Browman KE, Monk TH, et al. Napping and 24-hour sleep/wake patterns in healthy elderly and young adults. J Am Geriatr Soc 1992;40:779–86.

[20] Evans BD, Rogers AE. 24-hour sleep/wake patterns in healthy elderly persons. Appl Nurs Res 1994;7:75–83.

[21] Naska A, Oikonomou E, Trichopoulou A, et al. Siesta in healthy adults and coronary mortality in the general population. Arch Intern Med 2007;167:296–301.

[22] Monk TH, Buysse DJ, Carrier J, et al. Effects of afternoon "siesta" on sleep, alertness, performance, and circadian rhythms. Sleep 2001;24:680–7.

[23] Campbell SS, Murphy PJ, Stauble TN. Effects of a nap on nighttime sleep and waking function in older subjects. J Am Geriatr Soc 2005;53:48–53.

[24] Ohayon MM, Carskadon MA, Guillemenault C, et al. Meta-analysis of quantitative sleep parameters from childhood to old age in healthy individuals: developing normative sleep values across the human lifespan. Sleep 2004;27:1255–73.

[25] Van Cauter E, Leproult R, Plat L. Age-related changes in slow wave sleep and REM sleep and relationship with growth hormone and cortisol levels in healthy men. JAMA 2000; 284:861–8.

[26] Brandenburg G, Viola AU, Ehrhart J, et al. Age-related changes in autonomic control during sleep. J Sleep Res 2003;12:173–80.

[27] Dijk DJ, Duffy JF, Riel E, et al. Ageing and the circadian and homeostatic regulation of human sleep during forced desynchrony of rest, melatonin and temperature rhythms. J Physiol 1999;516:611–27.

[28] Wauqier A, van Sweden B, Lagaay AM, et al. Ambulatory monitoring of sleep-wakefulness patterns in healthy elderly males and females (greater than 88 years): the "Senieur" protocol. J Am Geriatr Soc 1992;40:109–14.

[29] Murphy PJ, Rogers NL, Campbell SS. Age differences in the spontaneous termination of sleep. J Sleep Res 2000;9:27–34.

[30] Crowley K, Trinder J, Kim Y, et al. The effects of normal aging on sleep spindle and K-complex production. Clin Neurophysiol 2002;113:1615–22.

[31] Nicolas A, Petit D, Rompré S, et al. Sleep spindle characteristics in healthy subjects of different age groups. Clin Neurophysiol 2001;112:521–7.

[32] Knoblauch V, Münch M, Blatter K, et al. Age-related changes in the circadian modulation of sleep-spindle frequency during nap sleep. Sleep 2005;28:1093–101.

[33] Smith JR, Karacan I, Yang M. Ontogeny of delta activity during human sleep. Electroencephalogr Clin Neurophysiol 1977;43:229–37.

[34] Darchia N, Campbell IG, Feinberg I. Rapid eye movement density is reduced in the normal elderly. Sleep 2003;26:973–7.

[35] Gori S, Ficca G, Giganti F, et al. Body movements during night sleep in healthy elderly subjects and their relationships with sleep stages. Brain Res Bull 2004;63:393–7.

[36] Monk TH, Reynolds CF III, Machen MA, et al. Daily social rhythms in the elderly and their relation to objectively recorded sleep. Sleep 1992;15:322–9.

[37] Münch M, Knoblauch V, Blatter K, et al. Age-related attenuation of the evening circadian arousal signal in humans. Neurobiol Aging 2005;26:1307–19.

[38] Cajochen C, Munch M, Knoblauch V, et al. Age-related changes in the circadian and homeostatic regulation of human sleep. Chronobiol Int 2006;23:461–74.

[39] Vitiello MV, Smallwood RG, Avery DH, et al. Circadian temperature rhythms in young adult and aged men. Neurobiol Aging 1986;7:87–100.

[40] Czeisler CA, Dumont M, Duffy JF, et al. Association of sleep-wake habits in older people with changes in output of circadian pacemaker. Lancet 1992;340:933–6.

[41] Duffy JF, Derk-Jan D, Lerman EB, et al. Later endogenous circadian temperature nadir relative to an earlier wake time in older people. Am J Physiol 1998;44: R1478–87.

[42] Bonnett MH. The effect of sleep fragmentation on sleep and performance in younger and older subjects. Neurobiol Aging 1989;10:21–5.

[43] Adam M, Retey JV, Khatami R, et al. Age-related changes in the time course of vigilant attention during 40 hours without sleep in men. Sleep 2006;29:55–7.

[44] Münch M, Knoblauch V, Blatter K, et al. The frontal predominance in human EEG delta activity after sleep loss decreases with age. Eur J Neurosci 2004;20:1402–10.

[45] Naifeh KH, Severinghaus JW, Kamiya J. Effect of aging on sleep-related changes in respiratory variables. Sleep 1987;10:160–71.

[46] Hudgel DE, Devadatta P, Hamilton H. Pattern of breathing and upper airway mechanics during wakefulness and sleep in healthy elderly humans. J Appl Physiol 1993;74:2198–204.

[47] Browne HAK, Adams L, Simonds AK, et al. Ageing does not influence the sleep-related decrease in the hypercapnic ventilatory response. Eur Respir J 2003;21:523–9.

[48] Sherman B, Wysham C, Pfohl B. Age-related changes in the circadian rhythm of plasma cortisol in man. J Clin Endocrinol Metab 1985;61:439–43.

[49] Kern W, Dodt C, Born J, et al. Changes in cortisol and growth hormone secretion during nocturnal sleep in the course of aging. J Gerontol A Biol Sci Med Sci 1996;51:M3–9.

[50] Prinz PN, Bailey SL, Woods DL. Sleep impairments in healthy seniors: roles of stress, cortisol, and interleukin-1 beta. Chronobiol Int 2000;17:391–404.

CLINICS IN
GERIATRIC
MEDICINE

ELSEVIER
SAUNDERS

Clin Geriatr Med 24 (2008) 15–26

Evaluation of Sleep Disturbances in Older Adults

Sumi Misra, MD, MPH[a,b,*],
Beth A. Malow, MD, MS[c,d]

[a]Assistant Professor of Medicine and Geriatrics, Division of General Internal Medicine,
Vanderbilt University Medical Center, Room A123 GRECC, Nashville Veteran's Affairs
Hospital, 1310 24th Avenue South, Nashville, TN 37212, USA
[b]Director, Geriatrics Primary Care Clinics, Tennessee Valley Health Care System,
Nashville Veterans Affairs Hospital, 1310 24th Avenue South, Nashville, TN 37212, USA
[c]Associate Professor, Department of Neurology, Vanderbilt University Medical Center,
Nashville, TN 37212, USA
[d]Medical Director, Vanderbilt Sleep Disorders Center, Vanderbilt University Medical Center,
1161 21st Avenue South, Room A-0106 MCN, Nashville, TN 37232-2551, USA

Older patients are at risk for a variety of sleep disorders, ranging from insomnia to circadian rhythm disturbances. The clinical consequence of unremitting sleep disturbances in the elderly population often includes hypersomnolence and may result in disorientation, delirium, impaired intellect, disturbed cognition, psychomotor retardation, or increased risk of accidents and injury. These symptoms may compromise overall quality of life and create social and economic burdens for the health care system, as well as for the caregivers. The clinical assessment of aging patients who have sleep complaints involves an in-depth multidisciplinary approach.

Sleep disturbances in older patients are common [1], multifactorial, and may contribute to increased use of health services [2]. Older patients are at risk for a variety of sleep disorders, ranging from insomnia to circadian rhythm disturbances. The clinical consequence of unremitting sleep disturbances in the elderly population often includes hypersomnolence and may result in disorientation, delirium, impaired intellect, disturbed cognition, psychomotor retardation, or increased risk of accidents and injury. These

This work was supported by the Geriatrics Academic Career Award from the BHPr.
* Corresponding author. Division of General Internal Medicine, Vanderbilt University Medical Center, Room A123 GRECC, Nashville Veteran's Affairs Hospital, 1310 24th Avenue South, Nashville, TN 37212.
E-mail address: sumathi.misra@vanderbilt.edu (S. Misra).

symptoms may compromise overall quality of life and create social and economic burdens for the health care system as well as for the caregivers. The clinical assessment of aging patients who have sleep complaints involves an in-depth multidisciplinary approach. The evaluation includes a detailed clinical history with specific tools (eg, the Epworth and Stanford Sleep Scales) as well as an overview of the objective assessment tools. Frequently used modalities include polysomnography (PSG), which is important in the assessment of sleep-disordered breathing, specific sleep stage abnormalities, nocturnal myoclonus, and unusual nocturnal behaviors. The Multiple Sleep Latency Test (MSLT) evaluates physiologic sleep tendency and provides objective assessment of excessive daytime somnolence. The use of electroencephalography during the PSG may be useful when evaluating patients who have abnormal nocturnal spells, such as rapid eye movement (REM) sleep behavior disorder (RBD) and nocturnal seizures [3]. In addition to these topics, this article includes a brief overview of the four categories of sleep disorders based on the international classification of sleep disorders.

Over the past few decades, research has shown that several predictable and normal age-related changes occur in sleep patterns and architecture (Table 1). These include sleep fragmentation [4], reduced sleep efficiency, decreased quality of sleep, and a decrease in restorative delta sleep by almost 2% per decade [4,5]. With aging, it becomes more difficult to fall asleep (increased sleep latency) and stay asleep at night, and more difficult to remain awake during the day. The absolute need for sleep does not decrease with age, but the ability to sleep does [6,7]. The total sleep time in

Table 1
Comparison of sleep characteristics in young and older adults

Young healthy adults	Older adults
Good sleepers	Increased fragmentation
7–8 hours in bed	10–12 hours in bed
Sleep 85%–90% of time	Sleep: 50%–70% of time
5% total awake time	25% total awake time
Less than 15 minutes to fall asleep	Greater than 15 minutes
Nocturnal awakenings few and brief	Multiple arousals and awakenings
Stage 1: less than 5%	Stage 1: 5%–10%
Stage 2: approximately 50% of sleep	Stage 2: 30%–50% of sleep
REM: 20%–25%	REM: 10%–25% (declines after age 65)
Stage 3 & 4: 25%	Stage 3 & 4: remaining 30%–45%
Summary of sleep patterns in healthy elderly individuals [12]	
Total sleep time reduced	
Sleep efficiency reduced	
Wake after sleep onset increased	
REM latency slightly reduced	
Delta sleep reduced	
Multiple sleep latency reduced	

Data from Feinsilver SH. Sleep in the elderly: what is normal? Clin Geriatr Med 2003;19: 177–88.

a 24-hour period appears to decline with advancing age [8], but a decrease in nocturnal sleep time is partially offset by increased daytime napping [4,9], with the prevalence of napping varying between 20% and 80% [10,11]. Although it is unclear whether the elderly need less sleep, nocturnal sleep does appear to decline with age. An expected feature of geriatric sleep is a decline in sleep efficiency: the ratio of time asleep to time in bed. This is mostly the result of multiple awakenings during the night, some of which can be prolonged. The latency to the first REM period decreases and the total amount of REM sleep may also decrease as a result of an overall reduction in total nocturnal sleep time [3].

In the elderly specifically, insufficient and inefficient sleep is associated with significant morbidity and mortality, decreased quality of life, increased depression and anxiety, difficulty with balance and ambulating, increased risk for falls, and subsequent increased potential for nursing home placement [13–15]. In comparison to matched controls, patients with sleep disturbances have slower reaction times, cognitive dysfunction, and memory impairment [16] which lead, to deficits in attention, short-term memory, decreased response times, and poorer performance levels [17]. In a longitudinal study of healthy seniors, decreased amounts of REM sleep and sleep efficiency were reported to increase the risk for all cause mortality, even after controlling for a variety of covariates [18].

Clinical evaluation of sleep in the older patient

A multifaceted approach is recommended in the clinical assessment of aging patients who have sleep complaints. The evaluation of a sleep disorder begins with obtaining a medical history focused on the chief complaint: the history of present illness, past sleep history, and past and present medication use (selective seratonin reuptake inhibitors, antipsychotics, cholinesterase inhibitors, anticholinergics), including timing and dosages. A detailed account of specific sleep complaints is necessary, with input from the bed partner, caregiver, or facility staff (for institutionalized elders). Excluding metabolic etiologies through a focused laboratory evaluation can help to guide the clinician toward the correct diagnosis. Initial screening should include panels for thyroid, kidney, liver, and hematologic functioning. Inquiries regarding lifestyle choices, such as smoking status, alcohol and caffeine intake, exercise, and sleep hygiene may reveal underlying causes for sleep disturbances. The following list addresses the various factors that can contribute to poor sleep in the elderly, which must be considered in the clinical assessment:

a) Many medical, social, and behavioral factors can contribute to poor sleep in the elderly (Box 1). The evaluation of sleep in this population also presents a unique challenge to the clinician, when compared with younger adults. Patients may lack the resources to make autonomous

---

Box 1. Common etiologies of sleep disturbances in the elderly

Lifestyle changes
   Retirement
   Change in residence
Napping
Medical illness
   Chronic cardiac disease (nocturnal angina, chronic heart
      failure, arrhythmia)
   Pulmonary disease
   Gastrointestinal (Irritable bowel disease, gastro-esophageal
      reflux disease)
   Endocrine (thyroid disease, menopause, diabetes related
      polyuria)
   Disease-related chronic pain (arthritis, neuropathy,
      malignancy)
Chronic renal failure
Medications and substances
   Diuretics (nocturia), anticholinergics, antidepressants
   Alcohol, caffeine, stimulant abuse
Psychiatric illness
   Mood disorders (depression, bipolar and dysthymic
      disorders)
   Anxiety (generalized, panic attacks, posttraumatic stress
      disorder)
   Psychosis (schizophrenia)
Primary sleep disorders
   Sleep-related breathing disorders (SRBD)
   Periodic limb movements disorder (PLMD)

---

decisions, appointments, or schedule procedures for evaluation and management, especially those residing in supervised care settings.
b) Co-morbid diseases confound the evaluation and testing process:
- Patients with arthritis have been observed to have problems initiating
  sleep (31%), maintaining sleep (81%), and tendency to awaken early
  in the morning (51%). Patients with rheumatoid arthritis have a high
  prevalence of restless legs syndrome (RLS) (25%) [19–21].
- Gastro esophageal reflux disease (GERD) is quite common with
  the general elderly population with, 44% of them having monthly
  and 7% having daily symptoms [22]. The relationship between disturbed sleep and GERD is bidirectional. Sleeping increases the likelihood of reflux, and reflux episodes often awaken the patient
  [23,24].

- More than 50% of patients with moderate to severe congestive heart failure experience Cheyne-Stokes respiration, increased sleep fragmentation, and an increase in daytime sleepiness [25,26].
- Diabetic patients have an increased prevalence of RLS, periodic limb movements of sleep, and obstructive sleep apnea (OSA) [27].
- [28] Patients on hemodialysis have a higher prevalence of OSA (which improves following dialysis), RLS, periodic limb movements, early insomnia, and excessive daytime sleepiness [29–31].
- Patients with dementia commonly experience disturbed sleep, with reports that 19% to 44% of community dwelling patients with dementia complain of sleep disturbances [32]. This may be a consequence of the dementia process itself, causing irreversible damage to areas in the brain responsible for regulating sleep. This theory is supported by the finding that those patients who have more advanced dementia, usually have more severe sleep disorders, in the form of daytime napping, abnormal nighttime behavior, wandering, confusion, and agitation [33].

c) Use of multiple medications: Medications in the elderly that disturb sleep via central nervous system activation include over-the-counter decongestants, beta agonists inhalants or oral formulations, corticosteroids and selective seratonin reuptake inhibitors (SSRIs). These medications have been shown to reduce sleep efficiency, delay sleep onset, and increase the number of nighttime awakenings. Specific drugs known to disturb sleep continuity include hypoglycemic agents, nicotine, alcohol, diuretics, and short-half-life hypnotics. Antidepressants, lithium, and antipsychotic medications exacerbate RLS and periodic limb movements.

d) Socio-economic barriers: Older adults are much more likely to have difficulty accessing medical services as a result of having inadequate transportation, limited social and financial resources, inadequate insurance coverage, and being homebound. Most elders have either Medicare or Medicaid coverage, which does not necessarily provide assistance in these areas.

Preclinical work-up

Sleep surveys

A variety of sleep questionnaires have been developed; one of the most well validated and widely used is the Pittsburgh Sleep Quality Index. This is a self-rated questionnaire that assesses sleep quality and disturbances over a 1-month time interval. Nineteen individual items are used to generate seven component scores: (1) subjective sleep quality, (2) sleep latency, (3) sleep duration, (4) habitual sleep efficiency, (5) sleep disturbances, (6) use of sleeping medication, and (7) daytime dysfunction. The sum of scores for these seven components yields one global sleep score [34]. This is a fairly lengthy survey and is most commonly used in clinical sleep research or in a comprehensive sleep evaluation clinic.

Another tool used primarily for research purposes is the Medical Outcomes Study Sleep Scale (MOS). The MOS was developed to study patients with chronic medical conditions. This 12-item subjective survey includes 10 Likert-type questions (score 1 = all of the time; score 6 = none of time) and two questions on sleep duration. The numerical scores are then transformed to a 0-100 point scale. The transformed scores are used to generate seven separate sleep scales: (1) sleep disturbance, (2) snoring, (3) shortness of breath or headache, (4) sleep adequacy, (5) sleep somnolence, (6) sleep problems index I, and (7) sleep problems index II.

A tool used for clinical assessment is the introspective measure of sleepiness, the Stanford Sleepiness Scale. This seven point Likert-type scale has descriptors ranging from "feeling active, vital, alert, or wide awake" (score = 1) to "no longer fighting sleep, sleep onset soon and having dream-like thoughts" (score = 7). The subject is instructed to choose the set of descriptors that best describe his feeling of sleepiness at the given moment [35,36].

The Epworth Sleepiness Scale (ESS) [37] is another simple tool used to subjectively quantify sleepiness using an eight-item questionnaire. Dozing probability ratings of zero (0), slight (1), moderate (2), or high (3) are assigned by the patient to eight hypothetical situations: (1) sitting and reading; (2) watching television; (3) sitting inactive in a public place; (4) riding as a passenger in a car for 1 hour without a break; (5) lying down to rest in the afternoon when circumstances permit; (6) sitting and talking to someone; (7) sitting quietly after lunch without alcohol; and (8) sitting in a car, while stopped for a few minutes in traffic. Based on reliability studies [38], one may assume that ESS scores of 10 or higher suggests chronic sleepiness. The maximum score is 24. Patients who have a total score of 10 or higher are often considered to have some degree of daytime sleepiness, and those with a score over 15 have severe daytime sleepiness [38]. The utility and validity of the ESS has not been tested specifically in older patients [39].

Given the limitations of the scales described above, in terms of use and validity in the elderly population, it may be more useful to use a direct and problem-focused line of questioning when obtaining a sleep history. In the elderly, especially in the nursing home population, questionnaires and sleep diaries are often difficult to administer given the frequency of comorbid cognitive and medical conditions. In these circumstances, a simplified sleep history is recommended which should include:

1. When do you wake up in the morning?
2. Do you feel that you are excessively drowsy during the daytime?
3. When do you fall asleep at night?
4. Do you have difficulties falling asleep?
5. How long does it take you to fall asleep?

6. How many hours do you sleep per night?
7. How many times do you wake up during a typical night?
8. Other questions pertaining to snoring, breathing cessation, and movements (kicking, twitching, or sensations such as creeping or crawling) in lower limbs
9. Narcoleptic symptoms (sleep paralysis, hallucinations at sleep onset or waking, cataplexy)

Caregiver input

Caregivers can frequently offer additional information regarding the patient's daytime functioning and propensity to fall asleep at inappropriate conversations or dangerous times (driving, operating machinery). Caregivers can also provide information that the patient is unable to provide, such as snoring, apneic spells, unusual nocturnal events, or nocturnal leg jerks. This "secondary information" is particularly valuable in elderly patients with cognitive impairment or inability to verbalize their sleep dysfunctions.

Post clinical information

The patient should be asked to keep a careful sleep diary for several weeks. This simple and inexpensive means of further characterizing the nature and severity of the problem can provide important therapeutic information [39].

Laboratory evaluation of sleep disorders in the older person

To understand the various objective testing modalities used in characterizing sleep disorders, the EEG activity during each stage of sleep is outlined below. Staging is based primarily on the frequency of EEG wave activity [40]. EEG activity includes beta activity (13 Hz), sleep spindles (bursts of 12 Hz–14 Hz), alpha rhythm (8 Hz–13 Hz), and theta rhythm (4 Hz–7 Hz), saw-tooth theta waves (4 Hz–7 Hz, with notched appearance), delta rhythm (0 Hz–4 Hz), and slow waves (12 Hz). Each 30 seconds of recording (1 epoch) is categorized as wakefulness (W); as sleep stage 1, 2, 3, 4; or as REM.

Sleep stages

- Stage 0 sleep is wakefulness (stage W or stage 0). The predominant EEG rhythm during eyes-closed wakefulness is alpha activity. Less than 5% of individuals do not have distinct alpha activity, for whom, alternative signs of sleep should be considered (eg, slow rolling eye movements).
- Stage 1 sleep is scored with a low-voltage, mixed-frequency EEG with no REM. Stage 1 sleep is a nonalpha state with EEG activity that has

neither delta nor slow waves; however, vertex sharp waves and slow rolling eye movements may be present.

- Stage 2 sleep is scored when there are sleep spindles or K complexes, but
  high-amplitude (75 micro-volts or greater) delta EEG activity totals less
  than 20% of the epoch duration.
- Stage 3 sleep is scored when an epoch contains 20% to 50% delta (or
  slow wave) activity.
- Stage 4 sleep is scored when an epoch contains greater than 50% delta
  (or slow wave) activity.
- REM sleep is confirmed when eye movements and muscle atonia accompany a stage 1 EEG pattern. Saw-tooth theta waves are distinctive and
  frequently accompany REM sleep. In addition to the above, a wide as-
  sortment of physiologic activities can accompany REM sleep.

Objective assessment of sleep

Polysomnography refers to the simultaneous recording of multiple physiologic parameters during sleep. Sleep is staged by monitoring brain waves
via electroencephalography (EEG, typically two channels), muscle activity,
(typically the chin muscles via electromyography), and eye movements (elec-
trooculography). This assessment is used to explore abnormal occurrences
during the patients' major sleep period, including the assessment of sleep related breathing disorders, specific sleep stage abnormalities, nocturnal myoclonus, and unusual nocturnal behaviors. The three features of breathing
measured during polysomnography are airflow, respiratory effort, and
blood oxygenation.

The indications for PSG as described in the American Academy of Sleep
Medicine (formerly the American Sleep Disorders Association) practice parameters [41,42] are summarized in Box 2 [43]. In the elderly population, the
complexity and intrusiveness of testing, and the need for specialized centers
when performing PSG can be a limiting factor in its usage, especially in the
nursing home and assisted living population.

Multiple sleep latency test

The best-validated measure of daytime sleepiness is the multiple sleep latency test. It is used to determine if there is evidence of excessive daytime
sleepiness or an abnormal tendency for REM sleep to occur. Sleep latency
is defined by elapsed time from lights out to the first epoch of any sleep
stage, including stage 1 sleep. Daytime functioning remains the only measure of the significance of these sleep changes in elderly persons. The
MSLT evaluates physiologic sleep tendency in the setting of an appropriate
sleep environment. Sleep latency is measured during four or five 20-minute
periods in a laboratory setting that provides "nap opportunities" presented

---

Box 2. Indications for Polysomnography

PSG is typically indicated for
Diagnosis of sleep-related breathing disorders
Continuous positive airway pressure titration for sleep-related
   breathing disorders
Obstructive sleep apnea documentation before laser assisted
   uvulopalatopharyngoplasty
Assessment of treatment results before multiple sleep latency
   tests for suspected narcolepsy
Violent or injurious sleep-related behaviors
Atypical or unusual parasomnias

PSG is not typically indicated for
Diagnosis of chronic lung disease
Epilepsy not related to a sleep disorder
Diagnosis or treatment of restless legs syndrome
Circadian rhythm sleep disorders
Depression
Uncomplicated and noninjurious parasomnias

From Olejniczak PW, McGuire SM, Fish BJ. A discussion of sleep. Prim Care Clin Office Pract 2004;31:149–74; with permission.

---

at 2-hour intervals throughout the day. The test is continued for 15 minutes after the first epoch of sleep to determine if REM sleep will occur. If sleep does not occur, the test is terminated at 20 minutes after lights out, and the sleep latency is scored as 20 minutes. More than 70% of patients with narcolepsy have a mean MSLT sleep latency of less than 5 minutes. The occurrence of REM sleep during two or more naps is considered highly supportive of the diagnosis of narcolepsy [44].

The MSLT provides objective assessment of excessive daytime somnolence. This test has been criticized, however, for testing the ability to fall asleep, rather than the ability to maintain wakefulness, which might be more relevant to daytime function. A modified version of the MSLT, the Maintenance of Wakefulness Test, instructs patients to stay awake and measures their ability to do so. Sleep latency measured in this fashion is significantly reduced in elderly persons, suggesting that they are more somnolent than the general population. Older adults tend to fall asleep faster during the day as compared with younger adults [44,45]. In the cardiovascular health study of 4,578 adults older than 65 years, 20% of participants reported being "usually sleepy in the daytime." Sleepiness was more common in those with depression, loud snoring, medication use for heart failure, and sedentary lifestyle, among other factors [46].

Electroencephalography

The use of EEG during the PSG may be useful when evaluating patients who have abnormal nocturnal spells, such as the REM sleep behavior disorder and nocturnal seizures. Other tests of sleepiness, such as pupillometry and evoked potential studies, are no longer in routine use [47]. In settings such as the nursing home, behavioral observation and actigraphy (an ambulatory activity-monitoring device that uses activity as a surrogate for wakefulness and rest as a surrogate for sleep) are good ways to study sleep because they are nonintrusive, feasible, and economical.

Summary

Although the elderly show an increased prevalence of sleep disorders and changes in both sleep architecture and sleep-wake cycles, disrupted sleep is not an inevitable part of aging. The aging process itself does not cause sleep problems and sleep requirements do not decrease with advanced age. The older person has lower "quality" sleep with increased fragmentation, less deep delta wave sleep, and tends to experience early morning awakenings. The prevalence of sleep disorders (dyssomnias, parasomnias, SRBD, periodic limb movements of sleep, and RLS) increase with age. When older patients have sleep disorders, they often present with excessive daytime sleepiness, insomnia, or abnormal motor activity.

In making the appropriate diagnosis, the medical provider must review the patient's medical history, psychiatric history, medications, underlying medical illnesses, and sleep-wake pattern. In some older adults, there are intrinsic limitations with certain testing methods based on the living situation, socioeconomic status, and underlying medical conditions. These factors must be considered when selecting the evaluation modality.

As many sleep disorders are potentially reversible and treatable, the primary care provider would be advised to screen for these problems. When a sleep disturbance is identified in the older adult, a thoughtfully evaluated, problem-based, clinical decision-making process can significantly improve quality of life and daytime function. In fact, the authors recommend that an assessment of sleep could be an integral component of the comprehensive geriatric assessment.

References

[1] Foley DJ, Monjan AA, Brown SL, et al. Sleep complaints among elderly persons: an epidemiologic study of three communities. Sleep 1995;18:425–32.
[2] Novak M, Mucsi I, Shapiro CM, et al. Increased utilization of health services by insomniacs—an epidemiological perspective. J Psychosom Res 2004;56:527–36.
[3] Yavidan A. Sleep disorders in the older patient. Prim Care Clin Office Pract 2005;32:563–86.

[4] Avidan AY. Sleep changes and disorders in the elderly patient. Curr Neurol Neurosci Rep 2002;2:178–85.

[5] Ohayon MM, Carskadon MA, Guilleminault C, et al. Meta-analysis of quantitative sleep parameters from childhood to old age in healthy individuals: developing normative sleep values across the human lifespan. Sleep 2004;27:1255–73.

[6] Bliwise DL. Review: sleep in normal aging and dementia. Sleep 1993;16:40–81.

[7] Ancoli-Israel S. Sleep problems in older adults: putting myths to bed. Geriatrics 1997;52: 20–30.

[8] Van Cauter EV, Leproult R, Plat L. Age-related changes in slow wave sleep and REM sleep and relationship with growth hormone and cortisol levels in healthy men. JAMA 2000;284: 861–8.

[9] McGee A, Russell S. The subjective assessment of normal sleep patterns. J Ment Sci 1962; 108:642–54.

[10] Prinz P. Sleep patterns in the healthy aged: relationship with intellectual function. J Gerontol 1977;32:179–85.

[11] Wauquier A, van Sweden B, Lagaay AM, et al. Ambulatory monitoring of sleep-wakefulness patterns in healthy elderly males and females (greater than 88 years): the "Senieur" protocol. J Am Geriatr Soc 1992;40:109–14.

[12] Feinsilver SH. Sleep in the elderly: what is normal? Clin Geriatr Med 2003;19:177–88.

[13] Barbar SI, Enright PL, Boyle P, et al. Sleep disturbances and their correlates in elderly Japanese American men residing in Hawaii. J Gerontol A Biol Sci Med Sci 2000;55:M406–11.

[14] Brassington GS, King AC, Bliwise DL. Sleep problems as a risk factor for falls in a sample of-community-dwelling adults aged 64–99 years. J Am Geriatr Soc 2000;48:1234–40.

[15] Tinetti ME, Williams CS. Falls, injuries due to falls and the risk of admission to a nursing home. N Engl J Med 1997;337:1279–84.

[16] Crenshaw MC, Edinger JD. Slow-wave sleep and waking cognitive performance among older adults with and without insomnia complaints. Physiol Behav 1999;66:485–92.

[17] Walsh JK, Benca RM, Bonnet M, et al. Insomnia: assessment and management in primary care: National Heart, Lung, and Blood Institute Working Group on Insomnia. Am Fam Physician 1999;59:3029–37.

[18] Dew MA, Hoch CC, Buysse DJ, et al. Healthy older adults' sleep predicts all-cause mortality at 4 to 19 years of follow-up. Psychosom Med 2003;65:63–73.

[19] Wilcox S, Brenes GA. Factors related to sleep disturbances in older adults experiencing knee pain with radiographic evidence of knee osteoarthritis. J Am Geriatr Soc 2000;48:1241–51.

[20] Salih AM, Gray RE, Mills KR. A clinical, serological and neurophysiological study of RLS in Rheumatoid Arthritis. Br J Rheumatol 1994;33:60–3.

[21] Jordan JM, Bernard SL. Self reported arthritis-related disruptions in sleep and daily life and the use of medical complementary and self care strategies for arthritis. Arch Fam Med 2000; 9:143–9.

[22] Locke GR III, Talley NJ. Prevalence and clinical spectrum of GERD: a population based study in Olmstead County, Minnesota. Gastroenterolgy 1997;112:1448–56.

[23] Orr WC. Sleep and gastrointestinal disease, A wake-up call. Rev Gastroenterol Disord 2004;(9 Suppl 4):S25–32.

[24] Foresman BH. Sleep related gastresophageal reflux. J Am Osteopath Assoc 2000; 100(12 suppl Pt 2):S7–10.

[25] Chocron S, Tatou E. Percieved Health status in patients over 70 before and after open heart operations. Age Ageing 2000;29:329–34.

[26] Perker Y, Hedner J. Respiratory disturbance index; an independent predictor of mortality in coronary artery disease. Am J Respir Crit Care Med 2000;162:81–6.

[27] Sridhar GR, Madu K. Prevalence of sleep disturbances in diabetics. Diabetes Res Clin Pract 1994;23:183–6.

[28] Lamond N, Tiggemann M. Factors predicting sleep disturbances in Type II diabetes. Sleep 2000;23:415–6.

[29] Williams SW, Tell GS. Correlates of sleep behaviour among hemodyalisis patients: the kidney Outcomes Prediction and Evaluation (KOPE) study. Am J Nephrol 2002;22:18–22.

[30] Parker KP. Sleep disturbances in dialysis patients. Sleep Med Rev 2003;7:131–43.

[31] Hanly PJ. Improvement of sleep apnea in patients with chronic renal failure who undergo nocturnal hemodialysis. N Engl J Med 2001;344:102–7.

[32] McCurry SM, Reynolds CF, Anconi-Israel S, et al. Treatment of sleep disorders in Alzheimer's disease. Sleep Med Rev 2000;4:603–28.

[33] Pat-Horenczyk R, Klauber MR, Schochat T, et al. Hourly profiles of sleep and wakefulness in severe versus mild-moderately demented nursing home patients. Aging Clin Exp Res 1998; 10:308–15.

[34] Buysse D, Reynolds C, Monk T, et al. The Pittsburgh sleep quality index: a new instrument for psychiatric practice and research. Psychiatry Res 1989;28:193–213.

[35] Hoddes E, Dement W, Zarcone V. The development and use of the Stanford Sleepiness Scale (SSS). Psychophysiology 1971;9:150.

[36] Mitler MM, Carskadon MA, Hirshkowitz M. Evaluating sleepiness. In: Kryger MH, Roth T, Dement WC, editors. Principles and practice of sleep medicine. 3rd edition. Philadelphia: WB Saunders; 2000. p. 1251–7.

[37] Johns MW. A new method for measuring daytime sleepiness: the Epworth sleepiness scale. Sleep 1991;14:540–5.

[38] Johns MW. Reliability and factor analysis of the Epworth Sleepiness Scale. Sleep 1992;15: 376–81.

[39] Morin C. Insomnia: psychological assessment and management. New York: The Guilford Press; 1993.

[40] Rechtschaffen A, Kales A, editors. A manual of standardized terminology, techniques and scoring system for sleep stages of human subjects. Washington, DC: US Government Printing Office; 1968. NIH publication no. 204.

[41] American Sleep Disorders Association Report. Practice parameters for the indications for polysomnography and related procedures: indications for Polysomnography Task Force, American Sleep Disorders Association Standards of Practice Committee. Sleep 1997;20: 406–22.

[42] Chesson AL, Ferber RA, Fry JM, et al. An American Sleep Disorders Association review. The indications for polysomnography and related procedures. Sleep 1997;20:423–87.

[43] Olejniczak PW, McGuire SM, Fisch BJ, et al. A discussion of sleep. Prim Care Clin Office Pract 2004;31:149–74.

[44] Dement WC, Miles LE, Carskadon MA. "White paper" on sleep and aging. J Am Geriatr Soc 1982;30:25–50.

[45] Dement W, Richardson G, Prinz P, et al. Changes of sleep and wakefulness with age. New York: Van Nostrand Reinhold; 1996.

[46] Whitney CW, Enright PL, Newman AB, et al. Correlates of daytime sleepiness in 4578 elderly persons: the Cardiovascular Health Study. Sleep 1998;21:27–36.

[47] Kushida CA, Littner MR, Morgenthaler T, et al. Practice parameters for the indication for polysomnography and related procedures: an update for 2005. Sleep 2005;28:499–521.

CLINICS IN
GERIATRIC
MEDICINE

ELSEVIER
SAUNDERS

Clin Geriatr Med 24 (2008) 27–38

The Effect of Chronic Disorders on Sleep in the Elderly

Aimée Dinorah Garcia, MD, CWS, FCCWS

Michael E. DeBakey Veteran's Affairs Medical Center, Baylor College of Medicine,
2002 Holcombe ECL 110, Houston, TX 77030, USA

Sleep is a basic biologic state that encompasses a large aspect of our lives, but it is not frequently discussed unless the individual begins having difficulties with insomnia [1]. Insomnia affects 20% to 50% of the adult population in Western countries, increases with age [2,3], and is reported more frequently in elderly women than in elderly men [4]. According to the *Diagnostic and Statistical Manual of Mental Disorders, fourth edition, text revision* (DSM-IV-TR), insomnia is defined as "difficulty in initiating or maintaining sleep or ... nonrestorative sleep" and as "causing clinically significant distress or impairment in social, occupational, or other important areas of functioning" [5,6].

Up to 57% of noninstitutionalized elderly people have problems with chronic insomnia [7]. This disorder can lead to significant morbidity, not only from the underlying lack of sleep but often from the medications prescribed in the treatment of the disorder [8]. In studies done on the effects of insomnia and aging, such as the Alameda Study and the Bronx Aging Study, correlation has been found between the number of hours of sleep and subsequent health and mortality. Furthermore, after controlling for depression, use of hypnotic medication, physical morbidity, age, and education, participants who reported longer sleep onset latencies performed significantly worse on measures of verbal knowledge, long-term memory and fund of information, and visual-spatial reasoning [9–11]. The impact of chronic insomnia is a decrease in overall function, both physically and mentally and an increased use of health care dollars. With the aging of the population, chronic insomnia will have an even greater impact on our health care resources [12–15].

Funding for this article was supported by a Geriatric Academic Career Awards, Health Resources and Services Administration, and the John A. Hartford Foundation.

E-mail address: aimeeg@bcm.tmc.edu

Change in normal sleep patterns with aging

Along with the physiologic changes that occur as individuals age, patterns of sleep are also altered. To understand abnormalities in sleep, it is important to understand the normal sleep cycle. The normal sleep cycle has three phases, which include light sleep, delta sleep, and rapid eye movement (REM) sleep. Light sleep and delta sleep are classified as nonREM sleep and are made up of four stages. Light sleep encompasses two stages (1 and 2). Stage 1 is the period between an awake state and early sleep, and stage 2 is the transition stage. It is during this phase that patients experience decreased heart rate, muscle relaxation, and decreased body temperature. Phase 2, which also has two stages (3 and 4), is known as delta sleep or deep sleep. It is considered the restful or restorative stage. The final phase is that of REM sleep. During this phase, which is the phase of active dreaming, patients exhibit rapid eye movement, increased heart rate, increased respiratory rate, and increased brain activity. Active muscle inhibition occurs to prevent the individual from acting out the dreams that occur [16].

Some of the most common changes with sleep in the elderly include a phase advance in the normal circadian cycle, decrease in the amount of delta sleep (phases 3 and 4), and a decrease in the total amount of time that individuals sleep [16,17]. In addition to the alteration in sleep patterns that have been described, changes in sleep can be caused by comorbidities that are common in the elderly.

Chronic illnesses affecting sleep in older adults

Changes that occur in all organ systems as individuals age may contribute to the development of chronic conditions. Many of these conditions are more prevalent in the elderly. Although the focus of this article is the effect of chronic disorders on sleep, in reality chronic diseases and insomnia are interrelated. Any physical illness that causes the patient discomfort can affect sleep, and the severity of the disease will naturally have a greater impact. Conversely, poor sleep quality secondary to sleep disorders have been shown to have effects on various chronic disorders. Some of the disease processes that have been associated with sleep disorders are chronic obstructive pulmonary disease (COPD), diabetes mellitus, chronic kidney disease (including end stage renal disease and nocturia), chronic pain, Parkinson's disease, dementia, depression, and malignancies [18,19]. The impact of these conditions on sleep is summarized in Table 1.

Chronic obstructive pulmonary disease

The prevalence, incidence, and mortality rates of COPD increase with aging up to age 85 and then stabilize or decrease; up to 10% of people aged 55 to 85 in North America have the disease [20]. COPD is the fourth leading cause of death in the United States, and the number of deaths attributable

Table 1
Chronic medical conditions impacting sleep

Medical condition	Impact on sleep
Chronic obstructive pulmonary disease	Reduction in arteriolar oxygenation
	Decline in baseline oxygen saturation
	• more frequent in "blue bloaters"
	• more pronounced in REM sleep
	Decline in ventilatory response to hypoxia
	Exaggerated breath to breath variability
	Exaggerated increase in respiratory frequency
	Sleep disordered breathing
	• hypopneas (partial respiration)
	• apneas (complete cessation of respiration)
Diabetes	Increased incidence of obstructive sleep apnea
	Increased incidence of sleep disordered breathing
	Autonomic neuropathy leading to ventilatory disorders
Dementia	Delayed sleep induction
	Prolonged wake time after arousal from sleep
	Increased activity during periods of wakefulness
	"Sun-downing"
	Increased day-time sleepiness compared with age-matched controls
	Exacerbated behavioral disturbances
Depression	Insomnia
	Increased number of awakenings
Chronic pain	Decreased sleep time
	Delayed sleep onset
	Increased nighttime awakenings
	Increase in depressive symptoms
Parkinson's disease	Decreased total sleep time
	Increased nighttime arousals
	Decreased sleep efficiency
Malignancies	Excessive fatigue
	Leg restlessness
	Insomnia
	Excessive sleepiness
Chronic kidney disease and incontinence	Restless legs syndrome
	Periodic limb movement
	Sleep apnea

to COPD is increasing [21]. In patients who do not have COPD, there are normal changes in the respiratory pattern during the sleep cycle. In the nonREM phase, there is a reduction in alveolar ventilation, a decrease in baseline oxygen saturation because of decreased arteriolar oxygenation, and a decreased ventilatory response to hypoxia [21]. During REM sleep, there is increased breath to breath variability and increased respiratory frequency [21]. There is also a continued decrease response to carbon dioxide when compared with nonREM sleep. These normal physiologic patterns are altered in patients with COPD. In addition to the physiologic changes described, there is also sleep disordered breathing (SDB), which is characterized by respiratory events that may include hypopneas (partial respiration) or apneas (complete cessation of respiration) during sleep. SDB is more common in older adults, with a prevalence of 45% to 62% in individuals over the age of 60, as compared with 4% to 9% in individuals between 30 and 60 years old [22]. SDB can be further exacerbated in those patients with concomitant COPD. Studies have shown that there is recurrent frequent hypoxemia in patients with COPD that is transient in nature, especially those who have the "blue bloater" phenotype [21,23–25]. This hypoxemia is exaggerated during REM sleep when there is respiratory muscle atonia. The result in a patient with COPD is increased nighttime arousals, sleep disruption, pulmonary hypertension, and increased overall mortality [26]. Wheezing and increased sputum production are positive predictors of difficulty in initiating or maintaining sleep [19].

Diabetes mellitus

The incidence of diabetes mellitus increases with age, in part because of age related changes in lean and fat body mass. The prevalence rates vary from 9.1% to 16.6% in individuals over the age of 65 [27,28]. The risk factors that are associated with diabetes mellitus, such as obesity, visceral fat storage, and age are also associated with sleep disorders, especially obstructive sleep apnea and sleep disordered breathing [29]. In addition to sharing many risk factors, both diabetes mellitus and SDB are associated with adverse cardiovascular outcomes, such as coronary artery disease, hypertension and coronary events [30–32]. Although studies have shown an increase in HgbA1c and impaired glucose tolerance as a result of SDB, there have also been studies that have shown an independent correlation between diabetes mellitus and sleep disorders [18,29,33,34]. Diabetes is also associated with autonomic neuropathy, which can lead to ventilatory disorders. A study by Ficker and colleagues [35] showed that 25% of patients with autonomic neuropathy secondary to diabetes had associated sleep apnea. This number was significantly higher than that for patients with diabetes mellitus without autonomic neuropathy. In addition to the respiratory effects, patients with diabetic neuropathy are also at higher risk of having urinary incontinence and pain, both of which are independent factors contributing to poor sleep.

Dementia

Dementia is a common disorder affecting the elderly, with an incidence of 30% to 50% in those individuals over the age of 85. Sleep problems in this population affect not only the patient, but the caregivers as well, and are a common cause of institutionalization [36–38]. Dementia subgroups include Alzheimer's-type, Parkinson's-related, fronto-temporal, and vascular dementia [39]. Alzheimer's-type dementia is the most common, affecting approximately 4.5 million people in the United States, and up to 44% of these patients are affected with sleep disturbances [39–42]. Overall, the dementias are associated with deterioration in the structure and the 24-hour distribution of sleep. Some common sleep problems with dementia patients include taking longer to get to sleep, staying awake longer when disturbed, tending to be more active during periods of wakefulness, and greater likelihood of sleeping during the day than age-matched controls [43,44]. In addition, when patients with dementia are placed in an institutional setting, this further affects overall sleep patterns [45,46]. Although daytime sleeping in community dwelling elders is associated with functional and cognitive impairment and future cognitive decline, in nursing home patients, insomnia and sleep disturbance are associated with increased mortality, but effects on quality of life are not well understood [47–49]. There are several factors that contribute to the problems with sleep in an institutional setting. Some potentially reversible factors are limited sunlight exposure, extended time spent in bed, physical inactivity, a disruptive nighttime environment (including noise and light), and poor sleep hygiene [50,51]. Dementia and snoring are the biggest predictors of disrupted sleep in nursing homes [52].

Depression

Depression is a common problem in the elderly. In patients over the age of 65, the prevalence in the community is 1%, and increases to 15% to 30% in long-term care facilities [53]. Risk factors for depression are a history of depression, chronic medical illness, female sex, being single or divorced, brain disease, alcohol abuse, use of certain medications, and stressful life events [54]. Unlike younger patients, the elderly typically present with less specific symptoms of depression, such as insomnia, anxiety, or fatigue [55]. In fact, insomnia is a defining feature of major depression in the DSM-IV [56]. Longitudinal studies have shown that the presence of insomnia predicts the subsequent onset of clinical depression, even when controlled for other potential causes of depressive symptoms [57–59]. In a study by Taylor and colleagues [60], elderly subjects with insomnia had greater depression and anxiety levels than people not having insomnia, and were 9.82 and 17.35 times as likely to have clinically significant depression and anxiety, respectively. Increased insomnia frequency was related to increased depression and anxiety, and increased number of awakenings was also related to increased depression [61].

Chronic pain

The prevalence of sleep disturbance among patients with chronic pain is high, and chronic pain and depression are closely correlated. A study by Sayar and colleagues [62] showed that depression causes sleep disruption in chronic pain patients, independent of pain intensity, pain duration, and anxiety. Approximately 50% to 88% of patients attending chronic pain clinics with nonmalignant pain reported that their sleep was impaired [63–66]. In the elderly, one of the most common causes of chronic pain is arthritis, including degenerative arthritis and inflammatory arthritis. A number of studies have shown a correlation between arthritis and insomnia, but these studies were small and focused only on the inflammatory type arthritis [67–71]. The prevalence of insomnia in patients with rheumatoid arthritis is 50% [71]. Predictors of greater numbers of these insomnia complaints included a greater number of involved joints, knee pain severity, cardiovascular disease, and poorer self-rated health, physical functioning, and physical performance [18,67]. Patients with high pain intensity reported less sleep time, more delayed sleep onset, and more nighttime wakening than did patients with low pain intensity [65]. The cycle that is created as a result of poor sleep causes may further increase pain sensitivity and thus lead to further sleep disruption, increased pain, and depression [72].

Parkinson's disease

Parkinson's disease is a common disorder affecting 1 in 1,000 individuals [73,74]. Sleep disorders are very common in Parkinson's disease because of the disease process itself and also the medications used to treat the disorder. The neuropathology of this disorder is known to affect anatomic structures and chemical neurotransmitters in the brain involved in sleep regulation [75,76]. The prevalence of insomnia in Parkinson's patients is between 60% to 98% [77–79]. The types of sleep disorders in Parkinson's patients can be divided in to two types: sleep disturbances and arousal disturbances. Sleep disturbances include light fragmented sleep, abnormal motor activity during sleep, REM behavior disorders, sleep related breathing disorders, sleep related hallucinations, and sleep related psychotic behavior. Arousal disturbances include sleep attacks and excessive daytime sleepiness [77]. When compared with age-matched healthy subjects, patients with Parkinson's exhibited a variety of sleep disturbances but most frequently a decrease in total sleep duration, likely because of increased nighttime arousals and decreased sleep efficiency. These disturbances are one of the potential causes of daytime sleepiness in this patient population [80]. A number of studies have shown that the factors that most affect quality of life in Parkinson's patients are depression, impaired function, and insomnia [81].

Malignancies

Insomnia affects up to 50% of patients with cancer, but has been under recognized as a cause of discomfort when compared with other symptoms, such as pain and fatigue. Insomnia and subsequent sleep disturbances can lead to fatigue and mood disturbances, with a profound impact on quality of life. It also contributes to immunosuppression, which may impact the course of the disease [82]. Insomnia in patients with cancer can occur secondary to pain, anxiety, and depression, or be a side effect of medications [83]. Physical and cognitive symptoms for people with poor sleep quality include tiredness, loss of concentration, low threshold for pain, anxiety, nervousness, irrational thoughts, hallucinations, loss of appetite, constipation, and being prone to accidents [84,85]. In addition to the physical problems caused by poor sleep, insomnia can also lead the patient to feel less able to cope with their diagnosis [86].

Oftentimes, the focus of the medical community is to treat the malignancy and the associated side effects from the medical therapies, such as mucositis and nausea, and issues of sleep are not addressed. In a study by Davidson and colleagues [87], a cross-sectional study was performed at a regional cancer center in Ontario, Canada. Patients from six oncology clinics were surveyed to determine the prevalence and nature of the sleep disturbances that they were experiencing. The most prevalent problems were excessive fatigue (44% of patients), leg restlessness (41%), insomnia (31%), and excessive sleepiness (28%). The most frequently identified contributors to insomnia were restless thoughts, worries, and pain or discomfort. This disorder appears to be prevalent in patients with malignancies and needs to be monitored and appropriately treated to maximize health benefits and quality of life.

Chronic kidney disease

There are many disorders relating to the kidneys that can exacerbate sleep disturbances in the elderly. Among these are nocturia, chronic renal insufficiency, and end-stage renal disease.

Nocturia was defined by the International Continence Society as "waking at night to void," and applies to any number of nighttime awakenings [88]. Nocturia is associated with aging and can result from behavioral influences (eg, late-night fluid intake, caffeine) or from several clinical conditions (eg, diabetes, congestive heart failure, lower urinary tract obstruction, prostatic disease, or overactive bladder) [89]. In one of the few studies in the literature on the effect of nocturia on quality of life and health, Koyne and colleagues [90] noted that there was an incremental effect on health related quality of life (HRQoL) and poor sleep quality, with increased episodes of nocturia greater than one episode per night. With increasing episodes of nocturia, the symptoms of "bother," affect on sleep, and HRQoL were further exacerbated. The overall effect was a total decrease in sleep, a significant effect on quality of life, and a greater need for medical care.

The effect of chronic kidney disease and sleep is not as well understood, but a study by Iliescu and colleagues [91] showed the prevalence of "poor sleep" in patients with chronic kidney disease was 53%, and was comparable to those patients with end stage renal disease on dialysis. Some of the factors thought to play a role in sleep disorders in chronic kidney disease include uremia [92–94], anemia, and iron deficiency, which have been linked to restless legs syndrome and periodic limb movement [95], and alterations in melatonin metabolism [96]. In addition, many of the medications used in the treatment of chronic kidney disease and end stage renal disease are known to affect sleep [97]. Once patients advance to end stage kidney disease, especially those on dialysis, the issues with sleep disorders worsens. Of patients with end stage renal disease on dialysis, 50% to 80% report sleep disturbances, which include restless legs syndrome, periodic limb movement, and sleep apnea. The most serious is obstructive sleep apnea, which has an associated increase in mortality in end stage renal disease patients. This has a significant effect on quality of life for these patients, especially when there is daytime disruption of activities because of fatigue and sleepiness [98].

Summary

As health care providers, we must understand the impact of sleep disorders on our aging population. Many of the chronic medical conditions that are so prevalent in the elderly have a significant impact on sleep, and affect overall well being and quality of life. In addition, the lack of restful or sufficient sleep further exacerbates the disease itself. Since each chronic disorder has its own specific impact on sleep quality, the effect of multiple chronic diseases on sleep disturbance is likely additive. Further research on the effects of chronic disease on sleep quality is needed. As clinicians, it is imperative that we recognize the impact that sleep disorders have on the health of our elderly patients and consider insomnia to be one of the more important geriatric syndromes.

References

[1] Hyyppa MT, Kronholm E. Quality of sleep and chronic illnesses. J Clin Epidemiol 1989;42: 633–8.
[2] Corman B, Leger D. Sleep disorders in elderly. Rev Prat 2004;54(12):1281–5.
[3] Monane M. Insomnia in the elderly. J Clin Psychiatry 1992;53(Suppl):23–8.
[4] Vitiello MV, Larsen LH, Moe KE. Age-related sleep change: gender and estrogen effects on the subjective–objective sleep quality relationships of healthy, noncomplaining older men and women. J Psychosom Res 2004;56:503–10.
[5] American Psychiatric Association. Diagnostic and statistical manual of mental disorders—text revision. 4th edition. Washington, DC: American Psychiatric Publishing; 2000.
[6] Benca RM. Diagnosis and treatment of chronic insomnia: a review. Psychiatr Serv 2005;56: 332–43.
[7] Foley DJ, Monjan AA, Brown SL, et al. Sleep complaints among elderly persons:an epidemiologic study of three communities. Sleep 1995;18:425–32.
[8] George CF, Baycliff CD. Management of insomnia in patients with COPD. Drugs 2003; 63940:379–87.
[9] Beloc N. Relationships of health practices and mortality. Prev Med 1973;2:67–81.
[10] Wiley J, Camacho T. Life-style and future health: evidence from the Alameda County Study. Prev Med 1980;9:1–21.

[11] Schmutte T, Harris S, Levin R, et al. The relation between cognitive functioning and self-reported sleep complaints in nondemented older adults: results from the Bronx aging study. Behav Sleep Med 2007;5(1):39–56.

[12] Walsh JK. Clinical and socioeconomic correlates of insomnia. J Clin Psychiatry 2004; 65(Suppl 8):13–9.

[13] Hatoum HT, Kong SX, Kania CM, et al. Insomnia, health-related quality of life and health-care resource consumption. A study of managed-care organisation enrollees. Pharmacoeconomics 1998;14:629–37.

[14] Kuppermann M, Lubeck DP, Mazonson PD, et al. Sleep problems and their correlates in a working population. J Gen Intern Med 1995;10:25–32.

[15] Leger D, Scheuermaier K, Philip P, et al. SF-36: evaluation of quality of life in severe and mild insomniacs compared with good sleepers. Psychosom Med 2001;63:49–55.

[16] Wolcove N, Elkholy O, Baltzan M, et al. Sleep and aging: 1. Sleep disorders commonly found in older people. CMAJ 2007;176(9):1299–304.

[17] Rajput V, Bromley SM. Chronic insomnia: a practical review. Am Fam Physician 1999;60: 1431–8 [discussion: 1441–2].

[18] Ancoli-Israel S. The impact and prevalence of chronic insomnia and other sleep disturbances associated with chronic illness. Am J Manag Care 2006;12:S221–9.

[19] Katz DA, McHorney CA. Clinical correlates of insomnia in patients with chronic illness. Arch Intern Med 1998;158:1099–107.

[20] Merck manual of geriatrics. Available at: http//www.merck.com/mrkshared/mmg/sec10/ ch78/ch78a.jsp. Accessed May 23, 2007.

[21] Mohnsenin V. Sleep in chronic obstructive pulmonary disease. Semin Respir Crit Care Med 2005;26(1):109–16.

[22] Cohen-Zion M, Ancoli-Israel S. Sleep disorders. In: Hazzard WR, Bless JP, Halter JB, et al, editors. Principles of geriatric medicine. 5th edition. Philadelphia: McGraw-Hill; 2003. p. 1531–41.

[23] Catterall JR, Douglas NJ, Calverley PM, et al. Transient hypoxemia during sleep in chronic obstructive pulmonary disease is not a sleep apnea syndrome. Am Rev Respir Dis 1983;128:24–9.

[24] Douglas NJ. Nocturnal hypoxemia in patients with chronic obstructive pulmonary disease. Clin Chest Med 1992;13:523–32.

[25] DeMarco FJ Jr, Wynne JW, Block AJ, et al. Oxygen desaturation during sleep as a determinant of the "Blue and Bloated" syndrome. Chest 1981;79:621–5.

[26] Gay PC. Chronic obstructive pulmonary disease and sleep. Respir Care 2004;49(1):39–51.

[27] Wilson PW, Anderson KM, Kannel WB. Epidemiology of diabetes mellitus in the elderly. The Framingham Study. Am J Med 1986;80(Suppl 5A):3–9.

[28] Manton KG, Stallard E, Liu K. Forecasts of active life expectancy: policy and fiscal implications. J Gerontol 1993;48(Special issue):11–26.

[29] Resnick HE, Redline S, Shahar E, et al, Sleep Heart Health Study. Diabetes and sleep disturbances: findings from the Sleep Heart Health Study. Diabetes Care 2003;26:702–9.

[30] Grunstein RR, Stenlof K, Hedner J, et al. Impact of obstructive sleep apena and sleepiness on metabolic and cardiovascular riks factors in the Swedish Obese Subjects (SOS) Study. Int J Obes Relat Metab Disord 1995;19:410–8.

[31] Kiley JL, McNicholas WT. Cardiovascular risk factors in patients with obstructive sleep apnea syndrome. Eur Respir J 2000;16:128–33.

[32] Nieto FJ, Young TB, Lind BK, et al. Association of sleep-disordered breathing, sleep apnea and hypertension in a large, community-based study: Sleep Heart Health Study. JAMA 2000;283:1029–36.

[33] Renko A, Hiltunen L, Laakso M, et al. The relationship of glucosetolerance to sleep disorders and daytime sleepiness. Diabetes Res Clin Pract 2005;67:84–91.

[34] Punjabi NM, Shahar E, Redline S, et al, Sleep Heart Health Study Investigators. Sleep-disordered breathing, glucose intolerance, and insulin resistance: the Sleep Heart Health Study. Am J Epidemiol 2004;160:521–30.

[35] Ficker JH, Dertinger SH, Siegfried W, et al. Obstructive sleep apnea and diabetes mellitus: the role of cardiovascular autonomic neuropathy. Eur Respir J 1998;11:14–9.

[36] Vitiello MV, Borson S. Sleep disturbances in patients with Alzheimer's disease: epidemiology, pathophysiology and treatment. CNS Drugs 2001;15(10):777–96.

[37] Hope T, Keene J, Gedling K, et al. Predictors of institutionalization for people with dementia living at home with a caregiver. Int J Geriatr Psychiatry 1998;13(10):682–90.

[38] Pollak CP, Perlick D. Sleep problems and institutionalization. J Geriatr Psychiatry Neurol 1991;4:204–10.

[39] Grossman H. Dementia: a brief review. Mt Sinai J Med 2006;73(7):985–92.

[40] Carpenter BD, Strauss ME, Patterson MB. Sleep disturbances in community dwelling patients with Alzheimer's disease. Clin Gerontol 1995;16:35–49.

[41] McCurry SM, Logsdon RG, Teri L, et al. Characteristics of sleep disturbance in community-dwelling Alzheimer's disease patients. J Geriatr Psychiatry Neurol 1999;12:53–9.

[42] Ritchie K. Behavioral disturbances of dementia in ambulatory care settings. Int Psychogeriatr 1996;8:439–42.

[43] Bliwise DL. Sleep in normal ageing and dementia a review. Sleep 1993;16:40–81.

[44] Van Someren EJW. Circadian sleep disturbances in the elderly. Exp Gerontol 2000;35: 1229–37.

[45] Ancoli-Israel S, Parker L, Sinaee R, et al. Sleep fragmentation in patients from a nursing home. J Gerontol 1989;44:M18–21.

[46] Jacobs D, Ancoli-Israel S, Parker L, et al. Twenty-four hour sleep–wake patterns in a nursing home population. Psychol Aging 1989;4:352–6.

[47] Martin JL, Webber AP, Tarannum A, et al. Daytime sleeping, sleep disturbance, and circadian rhythms in the nursing home. Am J Geriatr Psychiatry 2006;14:121–9.

[48] Manabe K, Matsui T, Yamaya M, et al. Sleep patterns and mortality among elderly patients in a geriatric hospital. Gerontology 2000;46:318–22.

[49] Dale MC, Burns A, Panter L, et al. Factors affecting survival of elderly nursing home residents. Int J Geriatr Psychiatry 2001;16:70–6.

[50] Schnelle JF, Cruise PA, Alessi CA, et al. Sleep hygiene in physically dependent nursing home residents. Sleep 1998;21:515–23.

[51] Schnelle JF, Ouslander JG, Simmons SF, et al. The nighttime environment, incontinence care, and sleep disruption in nursing homes. J Am Geriatr Soc 1993;41:910–4.

[52] Ancoli-Israel S, Jones DW, Hanger MA, et al. Sleep in the nursing home. In: Kuna ST, Suratt PM, Remmers JE, editors. Sleep and respiration in aging adults. New York: Elsevier Press; 1991. p. 77–84.

[53] Alexopoulos GS, Katz IR, Reynolds CF, et al. The expert consensus guideline series. Pharmacotherapy of depressive disorders in older patients. Postgrad Med 2001 Oct;1–86.

[54] Boswell EB, Stoudemire A. Major depression in the primary care setting. Am J Med 1996; 101:3S–9S.

[55] Birrer RB, Vemuri SB. Depression in later life: a diagnostic and therapeutic challenge. Am Fam Phys 2004;69:2375–82.

[56] American Psychiatric Association. Diagnostic and statistical manual of mental disorders. 4th edition. Washington, DC: American Psychiatric Association; 1994.

[57] Breslau N, Roth T, Rosenthal L, et al. Sleep disturbance and psychiatric disorders: a longitudinal epidemiological study of young adults. Biol Psychiatry 1996;39:411–8.

[58] Ford DE, Kamerow DB. Epidemiologic study of sleep disturbances and psychiatric disorders. An opportunity for prevention? JAMA 1989;262:1479–84.

[59] Riemann D, Voderholzer U. Primary insomnia: a risk factor to develop depression? J Affect Disord 2003;76:255–9.

[60] Taylor BJ, Lichstein KL, Durrence HH, et al. Epidemiology of insomnia, depression and anxiety. Sleep 2005;28(11):1457–64.

[61] Wilson KG, Eriksson MY, D'Eon JL, et al. Major depression and insomnia in chronic pain. Clin J Pain 2002;18(2):77–83.

[62] Sayar K, Meltem A, Yontem T. Sleep quality in chronic pain patients. Can J Psychiatry 2002; 47:844–8.
[63] Pilowsky I, CreUenden I, Townley M. Sleep disturbance in pain clinic patients. Pain 1985;23: 27–33.
[64] Atkinsoti JH, Ancotii-Israel S, Slater MA, et al. Subjective sleep disturbance in chronic back pain. Clin J Pain 1988;4:225–32.
[65] Morin CM, Gibson D, Wade J. Self-reported sleep and mood disturbance in chronic pain patients. Clin J Pain 1998;14:311–4.
[66] Smith MT, Perlis ML, Smith MS, et al. Sleep quality and presleep arousal in chronic pain patients. J Behav Med 2000;23:1–13.
[67] Wilcox S, Brenes GA, Levine D, et al. Factors related to sleep disturbance in older adults experiencing knee pain or knee pain with radiographic evidence of knee osteoarthritis. J Am Geriatr Soc 2000;48:1241–51.
[68] Lavie P, Nahir M, Lorber M, et al. Nonsteroidal anti-inflammatory drug therapy in rheumatoid arthritis patients: lack of association between clinical improvement and effects on sleep. Arthritis Rheum 1991;34:655–9.
[69] Leigh TJ, Hindmarch I, Bird HA, et al. Comparison of sleep in osteoarthritic patients and age and sex matched healthy controls. Ann Rheum Dis 1988;47:40–2.
[70] Dominick KL, Ahern FM, Gold CH, et al. Health-related quality of life among older adults with arthritis. Health Qual Life Outcomes 2004;2:5–12.
[71] Drewes AM, Svendsen L, Taagholt SJ, et al. Sleep in rheumatoid arthritis: a comparison with healthy subjects and studies of sleep/wake interactions. Br J Rheumatol 1998;37:71–81.
[72] Moldofsky H. "Psychogenic rheumatism" or the "fibrositis syndrome." In: Hill O, editor. Modem trends in psychosomatic medicine, vol. 3. London: Butterworths; 1976. p. 187–95.
[73] Tandberg E, Larsen JP, Nessler EG, et al. The epidemiology of Parkinson's disease in the county of Rogaland, Norway. Mov Disord 1995;5:541–9.
[74] Mutch WJ, Dingwall-Fordyce I, Downie AW, et al. Parkinson's disease in a Scottish city. BMJ 1986;292:534–6.
[75] Larsen JP, Tandberg E. Sleep disorders in patient's with Parkinson's disease: epidemiology and management. CNS Drugs 2001;15(4):267–75.
[76] Nauseida PA. Sleep disorders. In: Koller WC, editor. Handbook of Parkinson's disease. New York: Marcel Dekker, Inc.; 1987. p. 371–80.
[77] Askenasy JJM. Sleep disturbances in Parkinsonism. J Neural Transm 2003;110:125–50.
[78] Lees AJ, Blackburn NA, Campbell V. The nighttime problems of Parkinson's disease. Clin Neuropharmacol 1988;11(6):512–9.
[79] Nausidea PA, Weiner WJ, Kaplan LR, et al. Sleep disruption in the course of chronic levodopa therapy; an early feature of the levodopa psychosis. Clin Neuropharmacol 1982;5:183–94.
[80] Clarenbach P. Parkinson's disease and sleep. J Neurol 2000;247(Suppl 4):IV/20–3.
[81] Karlsen KH, Larsen JP, Tandberg E, et al. The influence of clinical and demographic variables on quality of life in Parkinson's disease. J Neurol Neurosurg Psychiatry 1999;66:431–5.
[82] O'Donnell JF. Insomnia in cancer patients. Clin Cornerstone 2004;6(Suppl 1D):S6–14.
[83] Mystakidou K, Parpa E, Tsilika E, et al. Sleep quality in advanced cancer patients. J Psychosom Res 2007;62(5):527–33.
[84] Carter D. In need of a good night's sleep. Nurs Times 1985;13:24–6.
[85] Closs SJ. Assessment of sleep in hospital patients: a review of methods. J Adv Nurs 1988;13: 501–10.
[86] Theobald DE. Cancer pain, fatigue, distress, and insomnia in cancer patients. Clin Cornerstone 2004;6(Suppl 1D):S15–21.
[87] Davidson JR, MacLean AW, Brundage MD, et al. Sleep disturbance in cancer patients. Soc Sci Med 2002;54(9):1309–21.
[88] Van Kerrebroeck P, Abrams P, Chaikin D, et al. The standardisation of terminology in nocturia: Report from the Standardisation Sub-committee of the International Continence Society. Neurourol Urodyn 2002;21:179–83.

[89] Weiss J, Blaivas JG, Stember D, et al. Nocturia in adults. Etiology and classification. Neuro-urol Urodyn 1998;17:467–72.

[90] Koyne KS, Zhou Z, Bhattacharyya SK, et al. The prevalence of nocturia and its effect on health-related quality of life and sleep in a community sample in the USA. BJU Int 2003; 92:948–54.

[91] Iliescu EA, Yeates KE, Holland DC. Quality of sleep in patients with chronic kidney disease. Nephrol Dial Transplant 2004;19:95–9.

[92] Molnar MZ, Novak M, Ambrus C, et al. Restless legs syndrome in patients after renal trans-plantation. Am J Kidney Dis 2005;45:388–96.

[93] Winkelmann J, Stautner A, Samtleben W, et al. Long-term course of restless legs syndrome in dialysis patients after kidney transplantation. Mov Disord 2002;17:1072–6.

[94] Hanly PJ, Pierratos A. Improvement of sleep apnea in patients with chronic renal failure who undergo nocturnal hemodialysis. N Engl J Med 2001;344:102–7.

[95] Benz RL, Pressman MR, Hovick ET, et al. A preliminary study of the effects of correction of anemia with recombinant human erythropoietin therapy on sleep, sleep disorders, and day-time sleepiness in hemodialysis patients (the SLEEPO study). Am J Kidney Dis 1999;34: 1089–95.

[96] Naziri ND, Oveisi F, Reyes GA, et al. Dysregulation of melatonin metabolism in chronic renal insufficiency: role of erythropoietin-deficiency anemia. Kidney Int 1996;50:653–6.

[97] Novak M, Shapiro CM. Drug-induced sleep disturbances. Focus on nonpsychotropic med-ications. Drug Saf 1997;16:133–49.

[98] Novak M, Shapiro CM, Mendelsshon D, et al. Diagnosis and management of insomnia in dialysis patients. Semin Dial 2006;19:25–31.

CLINICS IN
GERIATRIC
MEDICINE

ELSEVIER
SAUNDERS

Clin Geriatr Med 24 (2008) 39–50

Sleep Disturbances in Long-Term Care

Jennifer L. Martin, PhD[a,b],
Sonia Ancoli-Israel, PhD[c,d,*]

[a]Veteran's Affairs Greater Los Angeles Healthcare System, Geriatric Research, Education
and Clinical Center, 16111 Plummer Street, North Hills, CA 91343, USA
[b]University of California, Los Angeles School of Medicine, Multicampus Program in Geriatric
Medicine and Gerontology, 16111 Plummer Street (111), North Hills, CA 91343, USA
[c]Department of Psychiatry, University of California San Diego, 9500 Gilman Drive, La Jolla,
San Diego, CA 92093-0603, USA
[d]Department of Psychiatry, Veteran's Affairs San Diego Healthcare System,
3350 LaJolla Village Drive, San Diego, CA 92161, USA

A growing number of older adults reside in long-term care facilities. In this setting, residents commonly suffer from nighttime sleep disruption, which is often accompanied by daytime sleepiness and may be caused by a multitude of factors. Sleep disturbance is associated with negative health outcomes, including risk for falling, and elevated mortality risk among long-term care residents. A number of factors contribute to sleep disturbance in the long-term care setting, including medical and psychiatric illness, medications, circadian rhythm abnormalities, sleep disordered breathing and other primary sleep disorders, environmental conditions, and lifestyle habits. Based on research with older adults in the community and work conducted within long-term care settings, there is some suggestion that these factors are amenable to nonpharmacologic treatments. Further research on the broad implementation of treatments for sleep problems within the long-term care setting is still needed. Additional work is also needed to understand the administrative and policy factors that might lead to systemic changes in how sleep is viewed and sleep problems are addressed in long-term care settings.

Supported by NIA UCLA Claude Pepper Older Americans Independence Center (5 P60 AG010415), NCI CA112035 CBCRP 11IB-0034, M01 RR00827, NIA AG08415, and the Research Service of the Veterans Affairs San Diego Healthcare System.

* Corresponding author. Department of Psychiatry, University of California San Diego, 9500 Gilman Drive, La Jolla, San Diego, CA 92093-0603.
E-mail address: sancoliisrael@ucsd.edu (S. Ancoli-Israel).

doi:10.1016/j.cger.2007.08.001   *geriatric.theclinics.com*

As the number of older adults increases, the long-term and rehabilitative care needs of this growing segment of the population are often met in long-term care facilities. In 1999, approximately 5% of United States adults over age 65 resided in long-term care facilities. The typical long-term care resident is white (88%), widowed (63%), female (75%), and over age 75 (86%). Nearly all residents (97%) require assistance in one or more basic activities of daily living (eg, toileting, bathing, dressing). Residents are most commonly admitted from acute care hospitals (44%) or directly from their home (32%). The average length of stay in a long-term care facility is 2.4 years, and the most common reasons for discharge are death (27%) and acute hospital admission (28%), generally because of deteriorating health or acute medical emergency. Only 29% of residents are discharged because they recover or are sufficiently stabilized to return home [1]. Over 90% of long-term care residents receive nursing and medical services, assistance with medications, and assistance with personal care needs [1].

Sleep/wake patterns in long-term care residents

Nearly any visitor to a long-term care facility will see evidence of sleep/wake pattern disturbance among residents. Among long-term care residents, self-reported difficulties with sleep are even more common and more severe than among older adults living at home in the community. Residents are commonly asleep intermittently at all hours of the day, even during mealtime periods. Although older community-dwelling adults are more likely to take naps than younger adults, the typical long-term care resident shows a pattern of wakefulness that is frequently interrupted by brief periods of sleep. This daytime "wake fragmentation" is oftentimes accompanied by nighttime "sleep fragmentation." While it is impossible to determine which is causal and which is symptomatic, clearly nighttime wakefulness can lead to increased daytime sleeping, and vice versa. This vicious cycle can lead to extreme disruption of sleep/wake patterns. This is likely caused, in part, by changes in sleep associated with dementia, which is common in the long-term care setting as well (Table 1) [2].

Research using either behavioral observations of sleep or wrist actigraphy (an objective estimate of sleep, measured using wrist movements) has shown that the sleep of long-term care residents is distributed across the 24-hour day rather than being consolidated to the nighttime hours. Residents rarely are asleep or awake for a continuous hour during the day or night [3,4].

Some of the consequences of poor sleep, such as irritability, poor concentration and memory, slower reaction time, and decreased performance may all be assumed to be part of dementia. These symptoms, however, may also be a result of poor nighttime sleep and high levels of daytime sleepiness. For example, new research suggests that in community-dwelling older women, short sleep at night, poor sleep efficiency (percent of the night spent asleep),

Table 1
Changes in sleep and circadian rhythms in dementing illnesses

	Alzheimer's disease [2]	Dementia with lewy bodies	Parkinson's disease with dementia	Vascular dementia
Subjective sleep quality				
↓ subjective sleep quality			✔	
↑ time to fall asleep			✔	
↑ Daytime sleepiness		✔	✔	
Sleep architecture				
↑ awakenings	✔	✔	✔	✔
↑ light sleep (stage 1/2)	✔		✔	✔
↓ deep sleep (stage 3/4)	✔	✔	✔	✔
Δ REM sleep	✔			
24-hour sleep patterns				
↑ sleep/wake fragmentation	✔	✔	✔	✔
↑ daytime napping	✔	✔	✔	
Circadian rhythms				
↓ circadian rhythm amplitude	✔			
Delayed circadian rhythms	✔			

↑ = increase; ↓ = decrease; Δ = change.

and increased napping during the day are all associated with increased risk of falls [5], as well as increased risk of shorter survival [6,7]. Poor sleep has also been associated with negative outcomes in the nursing home setting [8].

Although the specific causes of sleep pattern disruption vary from person to person, there are several common causes of sleep difficulties in the long-term care setting. These include primary sleep disorders, medical conditions, psychiatric disorders, medications or polypharmacy, and circadian rhythm disruption. Environmental factors (eg, noise and light during the night, low daytime indoor illumination, little time spent outdoors), and behavioral factors (eg, physical inactivity, extended time spent in bed) also appear to contribute to the disruption of long-term care residents' sleep/wake patterns.

Primary sleep disorders in long-term care residents

No large-scale epidemiologic studies have been conducted to examine the prevalence of primary sleep disorders in long-term care facilities. One could assume, however, that sleep disorders that increase in prevalence with advancing age are at least as common among patients in long-term care facilities as in older adults in community settings, such as sleep disordered breathing (SDB), restless legs syndrome (RLS), periodic limb movement disorder (PLMD), and rapid eye movement (REM) sleep behavior disorder. In addition, these sleep disorders are even more common among individuals with certain dementing illnesses than among older adults without dementia (Table 2). The absence of true prevalence information in the long-term care

Table 2
Sleep disorders to consider in dementing illnesses

Illness	Sleep disorders
Alzheimer's disease	Sleep disordered breathing
Dementia with Lewy Bodies	Restless legs syndrome
	REM behavior disorder
	Periodic limb movement disorder
Parkinson's disease with dementia	Restless legs syndrome
	REM behavior disorder
	Periodic limb movement disorder
	Sleep disordered breathing
Vascular dementia	Sleep disordered breathing

setting is, in part, a result of the difficulty in conducting polysomnographic sleep recordings with long-term care residents, especially among individuals with dementia or extreme frailty.

Sleep disordered breathing is a condition in which airflow during respiration is interrupted. This can occur because the airway collapses during sleep or because central nervous system signaling is impaired. These respiratory events can involve a complete cessation of airflow (apnea) or a partial reduction in airflow (hypopnea). Events are considered clinically significant when they last at least 10 seconds and occur 15 or more times per hour of sleep. This can lead to decreased oxygen saturation and interruption of nighttime sleep. Both of these can contribute to negative consequences, such as increased risk for cardio- and cerebrovascular disease, cognitive difficulties, depression, and impaired performance. Depending upon the precise criteria used, one half to three quarters of long-term care residents have at least mild SDB. In the long-term care setting, research shows that SDB has been associated with cognitive impairment, agitated behaviors, and increased mortality risk [9,10].

SDB is generally treated with continuous positive airway pressure (CPAP). This treatment is not curative; however, it is highly effective in reducing the number of respiratory events. CPAP involves wearing a mask over the nose, which is connected via a hose to a machine that generates positive air pressure. This pressure acts as a splint to hold the airway open. While CPAP has not been evaluated for use with long-term care residents, recent findings suggest that Alzheimer's disease patients living at home with a caregiver have the same level of compliance with CPAP as general sleep disorder clinic patients [11]. The authors have observed some residents of nursing homes who used CPAP before institutionalization who choose to continue to use CPAP while in the nursing home. This suggests that CPAP should still be considered the treatment of choice among individuals in the long-term care setting who suffer from SDB, and residing in long-term care should not by itself preclude treatment of SDB [12].

Restless legs syndrome is a disorder in which an individual experiences an uncomfortable sensation in the legs while at rest. This discomfort, often difficult to describe, is relieved with movement of the legs. RLS symptoms often grow worse late in the day and can lead to difficulties falling asleep. RLS increases in prevalence with age, and individuals with RLS sometimes report that their symptoms grow worse as they get older. This condition has not been studied in long-term care; however, it may be a possible cause of motor restlessness and perhaps wandering among residents with RLS and dementia.

Periodic limb movement disorder is a related condition in which the legs jerk or kick during sleep. These movements can lead to fragmentation of nighttime sleep, which can contribute to daytime sleepiness. Treatments for both RLS and PLMD are pharmacologic and typically involve the use of dopaminergic agents. There are two Food and Drug Administration (FDA) approved agents for the treatment of RLS: ropinerole (Requip) and pramipexole (Mirapex). These agents have not been studied in the long-term care setting.

REM behavior disorder (RBD) is a condition in which the central nervous system mechanisms that cause muscle paralysis during REM sleep cease to function properly and the sleeper acts out dreams. In the long-term care setting, this condition has not been studied; however, RBD is most common among older men and among individuals with certain dementing illnesses (see Table 2). The main concern associated with RBD is patient safety. Individuals can fall out of bed or engage in dangerous behavior during the night as a result of acting out dream-related behaviors while asleep. The treatment of choice for RBD is clonazepam (Klonopin), which is effective in about 90% of patients. Treatment also involves securing the sleep environment to insure safety.

To date, no studies have systematically examined treatment of SDB, RLS, PLMD, or RBD in long-term care residents, and the safety and efficacy of these treatment, particularly among residents with severe dementia, is unknown. In general, treatment of primary sleep disorders in long-term care residents should closely parallel the treatment of frail older adults in the community. The risk/benefit ratio of each treatment should be considered. Key foci of treatment should be improvements in functional status, cognition, and quality of life. Clearly, further research on the treatment of primary sleep disorders in long-term care is needed.

Medications, medical illnesses, and psychiatric disorders

Long-term care residents are frequently in poor physical health: many suffer from dementia, depression, or both, and nearly all take multiple medications to manage medical and psychiatric conditions. On average, residents of long-term care facilities take five to eight different medications every day, and many take more than 10 medications per day [4,13]. Given that most residents use many medications, it is extremely likely that one or more of these medications impact nighttime sleep, daytime alertness, or both. Some specific medications can be particularly problematic when taken near bedtime, such as diuretics or stimulating agents (eg, sympathomimetics, bronchodilators). In addition, use of sedating medications during the daytime (eg, antihistamines, anticholinergics, sedating antidepressants) can contribute to daytime drowsiness, leading to daytime sleeping and further disrupting sleep/wake patterns. Some medications used in the treatment of depression, Parkinson's disease, and hypertension can impair sleep or cause nightmares as well. At times, changing the timing of administration of a medication can ameliorate sleep difficulties, particularly if sleep difficulties started or were exacerbated when the medication was first administered.

Residents of long-term care facilities are also likely to suffer from a number of medical conditions. Examples of common medical conditions among long-term residents that may contribute to sleep difficulty include pain (eg, from arthritis), paresthesias, nighttime cough, dyspnea (from cardiac or pulmonary illness), gastroesophageal reflux, and incontinence or frequent nighttime urination. While many of these are chronic conditions that cannot be treated directly, management of symptoms should consider both daytime functioning and nighttime sleep quality.

There is increasing evidence of sleep abnormalities with neurologic illnesses (eg, Alzheimer's disease, Parkinson's disease), many of which are common among long-term care residents. In the long-term care setting, residents are often in the late stages of these neurologic illnesses. Research suggests demented patients generally have more sleep disruption, lower sleep efficiency, more light sleep, less deep sleep, and perhaps less REM sleep when compared with nondemented older people (see Table 1) [14]. "Sundowning," the term used to describe a worsening of confusion and behavior problems in the evening or night in people with dementia, may have an underlying neurologic basis and is associated with circadian rhythm disruption [13]. The sleep abnormalities, excessive daytime sleepiness, and parasomnias (eg, REM sleep behavior disorder) associated with Parkinson's disease may be related to the pathology of the disorder or to its medication treatment. Problems may be even more common among long-term care residents with advanced disease [15].

Circadian rhythm disruption

Circadian rhythm disruption also contributes to sleep problems in long-term care residents. In older adults, circadian rhythms may be blunted in amplitude and can be shifted to abnormal times, and circadian rhythms are commonly altered among individuals with dementia (see Table 1). In one study, long-term care residents had less stable circadian rhythms of activity compared with older people living at home, regardless of cognitive status [16]. Other studies have found a relationship between circadian rhythm disturbance and degree of dementia [17]. Circadian activity rhythm abnormalities have also been associated with shorter survival in long-term care residents [18,19].

In addition to the often-cited advance (ie, shift to an earlier time) of circadian rhythms commonly seen in older adults, environmental factors also affect circadian rhythms in the long-term care setting. In particular, exposure to bright light is the strongest synchronizer and stabilizer of circadian rhythms, and daytime light levels in long-term care facilities are quite low, with residents seldom taken outdoors. Typically, long-term care residents are exposed to only a few minutes of bright light each day—even less than older adults living in the community [20]. Because light exposure is the strongest known "zeitgeber" (time cue) in human beings, this lack of daytime light may contribute to circadian disregulation. Long-term care residents also spend extended periods in bed and are physically inactive during the daytime which contributes to their circadian rhythm abnormalities. While physical activity has a weaker influence on circadian rhythms than light, it still plays an important role.

This disruption of circadian rhythms in the long term care setting contributes to fragmentation of sleep and wakefulness. This is because circadian rhythms exert a strong influence on the timing of sleep, and weak circadian rhythms or rhythms that are shifted to inappropriate times are likely to cause sleep problems. Circadian rhythm disturbances are best treated with timed exposure to bright light, and a number of studies have found that exposure to bright light strengthens and stabilizes circadian rhythms [21–23].

Long-term care facilities at night

Long-term care facilities are more similar to in-patient hospital settings than to home environments. Typically, residents share rooms, and the nighttime environment is not conducive to sleep because of frequent noise and light interruptions, which occur several times per hour, on average [24]. Long-term care residents must endure these interruptions on an extended, nightly basis. Research has shown that much of the noise produced in the facility is caused by staff, often while they provide incontinence and other personal care to residents [24,25]. In addition to noise, nighttime exposure to room-level light has the potential to suppress endogenous melatonin, disrupt sleep, and shift circadian rhythms [26].

Pharmacologic treatment of sleep problems

Extensive long-term care reforms enacted with the Omnibus Budget Reconciliation Act (OBRA) of 1987 (which became effective in 1991) included limits on the use of psychoactive medications in the long-term care setting. Although OBRA regulations specifically target antipsychotic medications, the interpretive guidelines that accompany these regulations also limit the use of anxiolytic agents and sedative-hypnotics, but not antidepressants. Use of regulated psychoactive medications must be documented in the medical record as necessary to treat a specific condition, with daily dose limits, requirements for monitoring treatment and adverse reactions, and attempts at dose reductions and discontinuation (if possible). The guidelines also provide options for using psychoactive medications outside of the stated limits when such use is clearly clinically indicated. Since the OBRA guidelines were implemented, research has shown substantial decreases in the use of antipsychotics among long-term care residents, with no change in the use of sedative-hypnotics or anxiolytics, and an increase in the use of antidepressants [27].

There are a number of FDA approved agents for the treatment of insomnia, and a number of additional medications that are commonly used "off label" to manage sleep problems. In 2005, the National Institutes of Health (NIH) State-of-the-Science Conference on Insomnia concluded that the newer shorter acting nonbenzodiazepine hypnotics were more effective and safer than older, longer acting benzodiazepines. In addition, the NIH clearly stated that all antidepressants have potentially significant adverse effects, raising concerns about the risk–benefit ratio when these medications are used to treat sleep problems in the absence of depression. Barbiturates and antipsychotics also have significant risks, and thus their use in the treatment of chronic insomnia was not recommended. In addition, there is no systematic evidence of efficacy and there are significant concerns about the risks of antihistamines (H1 receptor antagonists) when used to treat sleep disturbances [10]. The conclusions of the NIH panel were based primarily on studies conducted in younger and older adults, and not in older adults with dementia or those living in long-term care facilities. Although there are published reports on the efficacy and safety of the shorter acting nonbenzodiazepines in older adults in the community [28,29], research is still needed in the long-term care setting to establish the safety and efficacy of these newer medications.

When considering pharmacologic therapy for sleep problems among long-term care residents, it is important to consider the possibility that these medications can increase risk of some adverse outcomes. There are a number of studies that have found a relationship between the use of sleeping pills and falls [30–32]. It remains unclear however, how much of this relationship may be accounted for by the underlying sleep problems precipitating the hypnotic use in the first place. One recent study using administrative nursing home data in the Minimum Data Set (MDS) found that an indication of insomnia, but not an indication of hypnotic use, was associated with increased fall risk after controlling for many (but not all) fall risk factors documented on the MDS [33]. These findings, however, must be interpreted with caution because there are no data to support the accuracy of the insomnia or hypnotic use items on the MDS, and there is evidence that documentation of falls using this method is substandard [34]. Another important consideration is that nearly all prior work primarily included individuals using older-generation benzodiazepine medications. Research is needed in the long-term care setting to examine the safety and efficacy of the newer nonbenzodiazepines, and in particular, to examine the relation between insomnia and risk of falls versus use of these medications and risk of falls.

A second critical consideration is that, given the large number of medications long-term care residents already use, there is a potential for drug interactions or altered drug metabolism. Finally, use of pharmacologic agents for sleep problems should not be viewed as a substitute for addressing any other underlying causes of sleep disturbance such as, for example, sleep apnea, nighttime noise, inadequate control of pain, or circadian rhythm disturbances.

Nonpharmacological treatment of sleep problems

The NIH State-of-the-Science Conference on Insomnia also concluded that cognitive behavioral therapy (CBT) is as effective as prescription medications for brief treatment of chronic insomnia, with indications that beneficial effects of CBT (in contrast to those produced by medications) may last well beyond termination of treatment [35]. While it could be difficult to conduct CBT with patients with dementia because of cognitive limitations, several groups of investigators have undertaken studies to test the effectiveness of other nonpharmacological interventions to improve sleep in the long-term care setting, and have found some success.

Several studies have tested timed exposure to bright artificial light as a means of improving sleep/wake patterns. Bright light exposure impacts circadian rhythms. It can also increase alertness levels during and immediately after exposure. In randomized-controlled trials, long-term care residents exposed to bright light showed improved sleep relative to participants who received placebo interventions [22,23,36,37]. Researchers have also examined the effectiveness of supplemental melatonin (a hormone, typically secreted at night, that is closely linked to sleep), but results are mixed. Several aspects of the use of melatonin to improve sleep in long-term care residents, specifically, administration timing, dose, and preparation (acute versus sustained release) are not clear. A few studies have attempted to increase daytime activity levels, and results are, again, mixed. Some studies show sleep improves, while others show minimal or no changes in sleep [38]. Studies have also attempted to reduce nighttime noise and light in resident rooms. These studies have shown that it is extremely difficult to change the long-term care environment, and despite considerable efforts by researchers, the environment remains quite noisy at night [36,38,39].

An alternative approach is to use multicomponent interventions to address both internal physiologic causes of sleep disturbance and external environmental factors. One such study tested a short-term (5-day) intervention combining daytime light exposure and physical activity, a structured and regularly-timed bedtime routine, reduced time in bed during the day, plus provision of nighttime nursing care in a manner that minimizes disruption to sleep [36]. This intervention was successful in reducing daytime sleepiness, and residents who received the intervention were more socially engaged and physically active during the day than residents receiving usual care; however, nighttime noise and light were not significantly reduced, and there was minimal effect on nighttime sleep. There were also improvements seen in rest-activity rhythms with this intervention [21]. Significant improvements in sleep in the long-term care setting likely require that multiple factors be addressed simultaneously, perhaps for long periods of time (ie, weeks or months) in order for substantial improvements in sleep to be achieved and maintained.

One final area for intervention, which has largely been overlooked, is working at the facility level to change staff training, policies, and caregiving practices that impact resident sleep. The authors have conducted qualitative research in this area and have found that nightshift staff are well aware of the difficulties associated with disrupted resident sleep in terms of caregiving. However, many also felt that they needed to be busy during the nighttime hours, checking on residents regularly (often with lights on) and providing required nighttime care. The addition of sleep-promoting practices and the removal of unnecessary sleep-disruptive activities by staff may lead to meaningful changes for all residents in a facility. Real change will require administrators and other staff to buy into the notion that sleep is important and that encouraging better quality sleep/wake patterns is beneficial to both residents and staff over the long term.

Summary

In summary, nighttime sleep disruption is characteristic of long-term care residents, is typically accompanied by daytime sleepiness, and may be caused by a multitude of factors. Causal factors include medical and psychiatric illness, medications, circadian rhythm abnormalities, SDB and other primary sleep disorders, environmental factors, and lifestyle habits. There is some suggestion that these factors are amenable to treatment; however, further research on the implementation of treatments within the long-term care setting is needed. Specifically, further research is needed to determine whether treating SDB and other primary sleep disorders is feasible and results in functional or quality of life improvements among long-term care residents. Additional work is also needed to understand the administrative and policy factors that might lead to systemic changes in how sleep is viewed and sleep problems are addressed in long-term care settings.

References

[1] National Center for Health Statistics. Characteristics of elderly nursing home current residents and discharges: data from the 1997 national nursing home survey. Available at: http://www.cdc.gov/nchs/data/ad/ad312.pdf. Accessed September 12, 2007.

[2] Petit D, Montplaisir J, Boeve BF. Alzheimer's disease and other dementias. In: Kryger MH, Roth T, Dement WC, editors. Principles and practice of sleep medicine. 4th edition. Philadelphia: Elsevier Saunders; 2004. p. 853–62.

[3] Bliwise DL, Bevier WC, Bliwise NG, et al. Systemic 24-hour behavior observations of sleep and wakefulness in a skilled-care nursing facility. Psychol Aging 1990;15:16–24.

[4] Jacobs D, Ancoli-Israel S, Parker L, et al. Twenty-four hour sleep-wake patterns in a nursing home population. Psychol Aging 1989;4(3):352–6.

[5] Stone KL, Schneider JL, Blackwell T, et al. Impaired sleep increases the risk of falls in older women: a prospective actigraphy study. Sleep 2004;27:A125.

[6] Stone KL, Blackwell T, Cummings SR, et al. Rest-activity rhythms predict risk of mortality in older women. Sleep 2006;29(Suppl):A54.

[7] Dew MA, Hoch CC, Buysse DJ, et al. Healthy older adults' sleep predicts all-cause mortality at 4 to 19 years of follow-up. Psychosom Med 2003;65:63–73.

[8] Dale MC, Burns A, Panter L, et al. Factors affecting survival of elderly nursing home residents. Int J Geriatr Psychiatry 2001;16:70–6.

[9] Ancoli-Israel S, Klauber MR, Kripke DF, et al. Sleep apnea in female patients in a nursing home: increased risk of mortality. Chest 1989;96(5):1054–8.

[10] Cohen-Zion M, Stepnowsky C, Marler M, et al. Changes in cognitive function associated with sleep disordered breathing in older people. J Am Geriatr Soc 2001;49:1622–7.

[11] Ayalon L, Ancoli-Israel S, Stepnowsky C, et al. Treatment adherence in patients with Alzheimer's disease and obstructive sleep apnea. Am J Geriatr Psychiatry 2006;14:176–80.

[12] Gehrman PR, Martin JL, Shochat T, et al. Sleep disordered breathing and agitation in institutionalized adults with Alzheimer's disease. Am J Geriatr Psychiatry 2003;11:426–33.

[13] Martin J, Marler MR, Shochat T, et al. Circadian rhythms of agitation in institutionalized patients with Alzheimer's disease. Chronobiol Int 2000;17:405–18.

[14] Bliwise DL. Review: Sleep in normal aging and dementia. Sleep 1993;16:40–81.

[15] Friedman JH, Chou KL. Sleep and fatigue in Parkinson's disease. Parkinsonism Relat Disord 2004;10:S27–35.

[16] Van Someren EJW, Hagebeuk EEO, Lijzenga C, et al. Circadian rest activity rhythm disturbances in Alzheimer's disease. Biol Psychiatry 1996;40:259–70.

[17] Gehrman PR, Marler M, Martin JL, et al. The relationship between dementia severity and rest/activity circadian rhythms. Neuropsychiatr Dis Treat 2005;1:155–63.

[18] Gehrman PR, Marler M, Martin JL, et al. The timing of activity rhythms in patients with dementia is related to survival. J Gerontol A Biol Sci Med Sci 2004;59A:1050–5.

[19] Bliwise DL, Hughes ML, Carroll JS, et al. Mortality predicted by timing of temperature nadir in nursing home patients. Sleep Research 1995;24:510.

[20] Shochat T, Martin J, Marler M, et al. Illumination levels in nursing home patients: effects on sleep and activity rhythms. J Sleep Res 2000;9:373–80.

[21] Martin JL, Marler MR, Harker JO, et al. A multicomponent nonpharmacological intervention improves activity rhythms among nursing home residents with disrupted sleep/wake patterns. J Gerontol A Biol Sci Med Sci 2007;62A:67–72.

[22] Ancoli-Israel S, Martin JL, Kripke DF, et al. Effect of light treatment on sleep and circadian rhythms in demented nursing home patients. J Am Geriatr Soc 2002;50:282–9.

[23] Ancoli-Israel S, Gehrman PR, Martin JL, et al. Increased light exposure consolidates sleep and strengthens circadian rhythms in severe Alzheimer's disease patients. Behav Sleep Med 2003;1:22–36.

[24] Schnelle JF, Ouslander JG, Simmons SF, et al. The nighttime environment, incontinence care, and sleep disruption in nursing homes. J Am Geriatr Soc 1993;41:910–4.

[25] Schnelle JF, Cruise PA, Alessi CA, et al. Sleep hygiene in physically dependent nursing home residents. Sleep 1998;21:515–23.

[26] Boivin DB, James FO. Phase-dependent effect of room light exposure in a 5-h advance of sleep-wake cycle: implications for jet lag. J Biol Rhythms 2002;17:266–76.

[27] Lantz MS, Giambanco V, Buchalter EN. A ten-year review of the effect of OBRA-87 on psychotropic prescribing practices in an academic nursing home. Psychiatr Serv 1996;47:951–5.

[28] Ancoli-Israel S, Richardson GS, Mangano RM, et al. Long-term use of sedative hypnotics in older patients with insomnia. Sleep Med 2005;6:107–13.

[29] Contronco A, Gareri P, Lacava R, et al. Use of zolpidem in over 75-year-old patients with sleep disorders and comorbidities. Arch Gerontol Geriatr 2004;9:93–6.

[30] Campbell AJ, Borrie MJ, Spears GF. Risk factors for falls in a community-based prospective study of people 70 years and older. J Gerontol 1989;44(4):M112–7.

[31] Ray WA, Thapa PB, Gideon P. Benzodiazepines and the risk of falls in nursing home residents. J Am Geriatr Soc 2000;48:682–5.

[32] Schneeweiss S, Wang PS. Claims data studies of sedative-hypnotics and hip fractures in older people: exploring residual confounding using survey information. J Am Geriatr Soc 2005;53: 948–54.

[33] Avidan AY, Fries BE, James ML, et al. Insomnia and hypnotic use, recorded in the minimum data set, as predictors of falls and hip fractures in Michigan nursing homes. J Am Geriatr Soc 2005;53:955–62.

[34] Martin JL, Alessi CA. Limited validity of MDS items on sleep and hypnotic use in predicting falls and hip fracture among nursing home residents. J Am Geriatr Soc 2006;54:1150–2.

[35] National Institutes of Health. Manifestations and management of chronic insomnia in adults. Sleep 2005;28:1049–57.

[36] Alessi CA, Martin JL, Webber AP, et al. Randomized controlled trial of a nonpharmacological intervention to improve abnormal sleep/wake patterns in nursing home residents. J Am Geriatr Soc 2005;53:619–26.

[37] Van Someren EJW, Kessler A, Mirmiran M, et al. Indirect bright light improves circadian rest-activity rhythm disturbances in demented patients. Biol Psychiatry 1997;41:955–63.

[38] Alessi CA, Yoon EJ, Schnelle JF, et al. A randomized trial of a combined physical activity and environmental intervention in nursing home residents: do sleep and agitation improve? J Am Geriatr Soc 1999;47:784–91.

[39] Schnelle JF, Alessi CA, Al-Samarrai NR, et al. The nursing home at night: effects of an intervention on noise, light and sleep. J Am Geriatr Soc 1999;47:430–8.

ELSEVIER
SAUNDERS

CLINICS IN
GERIATRIC
MEDICINE

Clin Geriatr Med 24 (2008) 51–67

Insomnia Among Hospitalized Older Persons

Joseph H. Flaherty, MD[a,b,*]

[a]Geriatric Research, Education and Clinical Center, St. Louis Veteran's Affairs
Medical Center, St. Louis, MO, USA
[b]Department of Internal Medicine & Division of Geriatrics, Saint Louis University School
of Medicine, 1402 S. Grand Boulevard, Room M238, St. Louis, MO 63104, USA

Importance of sleep and consequences of sleep deprivation

When we are ill, the thought of restful sleep is paramount in our minds. The paradox is that it is as if the body is telling the brain to "heal, I need you to fall asleep," while the brain is yelling at our body, "I know, I know, if I could fall asleep, I would feel better too." This struggle becomes obvious when one examines the definition of sleep as "a natural occurrence having a psychological and physiological function that activates the restorative repair process of the body" [1]. How unfortunate, ironic, and iniquitous it is, however, that the location with one of the highest rates of sleep disturbances is also the place where most inhabitants are ill: the hospital.

The importance of sleep is evident from associations of sleep deprivation or sleep disturbances with a variety of negative outcomes: abnormalities in the hypothalamic-pituitary-adrenal axis [2], impaired healing of damaged tissues [3], impaired protein synthesis and decreased cellular immunity [4], cognitive impairment, including delirium [5], and even higher mortality. In one study of 272 older people in a skilled-care geriatric hospital in Japan, investigators observed patients for sleep disturbances hourly at night during a 2-week period. After adjusting for age, gender, and activities of daily living status, the presence of nighttime insomnia and sleep-onset delay was associated with a higher risk of mortality during a 2-year follow up period [6].

The high prevalence of insomnia and sleep disturbances among older hospitalized patients is obvious when one examines the use of sedative-hypnotic drugs. On general medical wards, 31% to 41% of patients receive these

* Department of Internal Medicine & Division of Geriatrics, Saint Louis University School of Medicine, 1402 S. Grand Boulevard, Room M238, St. Louis, MO 63104.
E-mail address: flaherty@slu.edu

0749-0690/08/$ - see front matter © 2008 Elsevier Inc. All rights reserved.
doi:10.1016/j.cger.2007.08.012   geriatric.theclinics.com

types of drugs. On surgical wards, 83% to 96% of patients are prescribed these drugs, and 33% to 88% of patients receive them [7–10]. These drugs are not benign, as they are associated with delirium, falls, hip fractures, dependency, and rebound insomnia [11–15].

Patients with certain medical conditions may have higher than average rates of sleep disturbances. For example, patients with Alzheimer's type or other types of dementia are at increased risk for sleep disturbances in the hospital if they have impaired sensory perception or have difficulty communicating their needs [16]. The prevalence among patients undergoing coronary artery bypass graft (CABG) surgery is particularly high, and this problem often persists. From 39% to 69% of patients during the first few weeks after hospital discharge have sleep problems, which can continue weeks and months into recovery [17–19]. In one study using a telephone survey, 68% of patients who had undergone CABG reported sleep disturbances at 6 months [20].

Secondary disorders and sleep disturbances

Although the emphasis of this article is on insomnia, the phrase "sleep disturbance" has also been used to give a broader scope to the problems that can occur and that can be identified. Queries about the quantity and quality of sleep, about the subjective and objective patterns of sleep, should be part of the standard medical evaluation of older patients. When something is amiss, it may represent an opportunity to identify or diagnose a treatable or reversible problem.

In one study, where researchers administered a questionnaire to over 200 patients with a mean age of 60 years, admitted to a hospital, 47% were found to have either insomnia, excessive daytime somnolence, or both. Over 20% of the total group had either restless legs or a combination of leg jerks and leg kicking. When the medical charts were reviewed, none had any documentation of complaints related to sleep [21]. Based on other studies as well, the hospital may be a good place to diagnose sleep disorders, such as sleep apnea or hypopnea (hypoventilation) [22].

Sleep disturbances among older hospitalized patients should also alert physicians and others of an underlying medical problem. One easy rule of thumb to remember is that if the nurses are requesting something to help the patient sleep, but the patient is not requesting something, then there is more likely a secondary cause of the insomnia. Delirium is one of the most common reasons that nurses call physicians at night, although nurses may not use the term delirium. They may say, "the patient won't go to sleep" or "won't stay in bed." They may say that the (delirious) patient is keeping other patients awake at night. It is difficult to care for delirious patients if there are fewer staff at night, and so a sedative is often seen as a solution.

Delirium is a diagnostic term for a clinical syndrome caused by either underlying medical illnesses (often presenting atypically as confusion) or medications. If the causes of the delirium are identified in a timely fashion, they can be treated, and the delirium will resolve in the majority of cases. As noted in the diagnostic criteria, according to the Diagnostic and Statistical Manual of Mental Disorders, fourth edition, sleep problems are part of the syndrome: "a sudden onset of impaired attention, disorganized thinking or incoherent speech, clouded consciousness, perceptual disturbances, sleep-wake cycle problems, psychomotor agitation or lethargy, and disorientation" [23]. Among hospitalized older patients, up to 22% have delirium on admission and up to 31% develop delirium while hospitalized. Even higher rates are found among orthopedic surgical patients and patients in the intensive care unit [24–28]. Physicians fail to recognize delirium in 32% to 66% of patients, and nurses in up to 69% of patients, oftentimes considering it just part of the hospital course [29–32]. Misdiagnosis or late diagnosis partly explains why delirium is associated with adverse outcomes [33], such as decline in physical function, increased hospital length of stay, increased discharge to a long-term care facility, and increased hospital costs [34–42]. Thus, when the call comes in the form of "the patient won't sleep," this should be considered an opportunity to make the diagnosis of delirium and find the underlying medical problem or medication causing the delirium.

Insomnia may also be a marker for serious underlying psychiatric disorders. In a review by Vitiello [43], as many as 50% of older persons with depression have sleep disturbances. In one study of 200 hospitalized patients, 56.5% complained of insomnia, and 50% suffered from at least one psychiatric disorder. Major depressive episode ($P < .001$), generalized anxiety disorder ($P = .025$), and suicide risk ($P = .034$) were associated with insomnia (univariate analysis). The results of the multivariate analysis showed that only a major depressive episode had a statistically significant association with insomnia (odds ratio = 3.6; 95% confidence interval [CI], = 1.9–6.9) [44].

Causes of insomnia

The causes of insomnia among hospitalized older persons are numerous and varied. They can be categorized as intrinsic or extrinsic to the patient (Box 1). Most causes in both categories are modifiable and treatable.

Intrinsic causes

Older hospitalized patients are particularly vulnerable to sleep deprivation for several reasons. Certain changes in sleep patterns are more common among older people, compared with younger, many of which can be amplified by the hospitalization. Older people may have more difficulty falling asleep, may have more frequent awakenings, and may be more easily aroused from sleep by noise or other environmental stimuli [45].

Box 1. Causes of insomnia among hospitalized older patients

Intrinsic
Changes in sleep pattern, which are more common in elderly
Underlying medical illnesses, such as delirium
Medications
    Clonidine, corticosteroids, bronchodilators, levodopa,
        leuprolide, phenytoin, pseudoephedrine, theophylline, and
        antidepressants such as buproprion, serotonin reuptake
        inhibitors, and venlafexine
Medication withdrawal
Alcohol withdrawal

Extrinsic
Hospital environment, especially for cognitively impaired
Patient care activities and interactions
Medication passes, phlebotomy, vital signs
Temperature
Light
Noise
    Staff conversation, number of staff, television, alarms,
        telephones, nursing call system, paging system, deliveries
        to floor, through traffic
Medical technology and monitoring
    Telemetry, intravenous tubing, intermittent pneumatic
        compression devices
Other patients

Medical illnesses may be the underlying cause of sleep disturbances or sleep deprivation. It is up to the astute clinician to determine if the telephone call from the nurse for insomnia is a clue that something is wrong with the patient. At the least, clinicians should ask for a set of vital signs, including the fifth (pain) [46] and sixth (mental status) vital signs [47].

In addition to the common medical illnesses, such as congestive heart failure, chronic obstructive pulmonary disease, gastrointestinal reflux disease, and benign prostatic hypertophy, subtle problems, such as pain in patients who cannot communicate well, urinary retention or incontinence, and delirium should be considered.

"Sundowning" is an overused and oftentimes inappropriate term used to describe older patients, usually with dementia, who have worsening of their confusion as the sun goes down and it becomes dark. If the term is used in this way, health care personnel are more likely to consider this expected, and pursuit of underlying causes may be ignored. The more appropriate approach to this problem is to consider this the onset or exacerbation of delirium during the evening or night [48]. In this way, physicians and others are prompted to identify underlying and potentially reversible causes.

Certain medications may cause or contribute to sleep disturbances. The most commonly used medications that may cause insomnia in hospitalized older patients are clonidine, corticosteroids, bronchodilators, levodopa, leuprolide, phenytoin, pseudoephedrine, theophylline, and antidepressants such as buproprion, serotonin reuptake inhibitors (SSRIs), and venlafexine [49,50].

One of the common mistakes clinicians make that leads to sleep disturbance is to order diuretics twice a day. In a typical hospital, this medication will be given at 9:00 AM and 9:00 PM. Similarly, orders such as "every 6 hours" may cause interruptions at night, because the medication will be given at 6:00 AM, 12:00 PM, 6:00 PM, and 12:00 AM.

Medication withdrawal, for example from benzodiazepines and even SSRIs, can cause anxiety, insomnia, and even delirium. Insomnia may be one of the first symptoms of alcohol withdrawal, which is considered a serious medical problem. Assessment tools exist for alcohol withdrawal and should be standard of care in hospitals [51,52].

Extrinsic causes

One of the common themes to keep in mind, as extrinsic causes are reviewed, is that although they seem like obvious reasons for sleep disturbances, the challenge for health care professionals is not to become desensitized to them. When people who work in hospitals are able to ignore the following or accept the following as "normal," then that is a signal that desensitization has happened.

The general hospital environment is an unfamiliar place to most people. This is an especially important point to remember for older persons with cognitive impairment, who may depend on routines and familiar objects to keep what little orientation they have, intact. Interruptions in the form of patient care activities or interactions of any sort occurring at night can disrupt sleep. The most common nighttime interruptions are phlebotomy, medication administration, and the taking of vital signs.

Room temperature may be a factor in sleep disturbances. Older people have less subcutaneous fat, thus may feel colder than staff who may feel comfortable at the hospital temperature. Evidence of this is discussed below under the interventions section, in which warm blankets were the most commonly requested item in a multicomponent intervention to improve sleep. Staff who are active or busy may even feel warm, leading a hospital's acceptable temperature to be based on how the staff feels instead of how patients feel.

Light

Light: the right kind, the right amount, and at the right time. All are important. Lack of diurnal light cycles may affect normal sleep function in healthy people, let alone those who are ill. Artificial light exposure for as little as 20 minutes during a normal sleep cycle can cause a drop in melatonin levels, and constant lighting can lead to a complete disruption of the normal melatonin concentration rhythm [53]. Melatonin not only facilitates sleep, but plays a role in modulation of corticosteroid and thyroid hormone levels [54].

Noise is a major factor in sleep disturbance and sleep deprivation in the hospital. Patients identified noise as the most important irritant after surgery in one study [55]. The United States Environmental Protection Agency recommends a maximum of 45 decibels (dBA) throughout the day and 35 dBA at night. However, most hospitals have noise levels from 50 dBA to 70 dBA during the day and an average of 67 dBA at night [56]. Noise comes in a variety of noticeable and subtle forms. Television, telephones, and alarms are the obvious forms of noise, but have potential to get overlooked as necessary or just part of the hospital environment. Anyone who has sat at a nurses' station realizes the noise levels from staff conversation. Although noise is a seemingly necessary part of hospital care, one study proved the obvious: there was a positive relationship between the number of staff present and the level of noise recorded [57]. Subtle sound pollution includes some nurse call systems, overhead paging systems, deliveries to the floor, and through traffic.

Medical technology is not only overused in some circumstances, but encouraged by our system of reimbursement, which is partially based on what we are "doing" to the patient. For example, intravenous fluids, at certain rates, are one of the main criteria for hospital admission, as are intravenous medications. Timing of these can disrupt sleep. Telemetry is another example of technology that is often used without clear necessity, and one that is often forgotten about after it is ordered. Intermittent pneumatic compression devices, while useful in some [58] but not all patient populations [59], to prevent deep venous thomboses from developing, are another cause of sleep disturbance among hospitalized patients.

Although no studies have looked at rates of insomnia among patients in semiprivate compared with private hospital rooms, this may be a moot point, as almost all new hospitals being built will have only private rooms. This is in part because of a directive, approved by the Health Guidelines Revision Committee, a 125-member committee of architects, developers, hospital administrators, engineers, physicians and facilities managers, which says that "the maximum number of beds per room shall be one" unless the facility can demonstrate the "necessity of a two-bed arrangement" [60,61].

The intensive care unit

One of the most studied areas of the hospital related to sleep disturbance is the Intensive Care Unit (ICU). Although everything noted above in this section applies to the ICU environment, some special remarks are needed.

The ICUs are one of the nosiest and busiest locations in hospitals. While several studies have shown that noise levels and patient care activities by nurses and other staff are so high that sleep disturbances seem unavoidable, results of two studies using polysomnography (PSG) monitoring suggest that ICU patients are qualitatively, but possibly not quantitatively sleep deprived.

In one study, researchers put sound meters at the head of an ICU patient's bed. The mean sound level was 84 dBA [62]. While there are many sources of noise, such as telephones, televisions, ventilators, alarms, and staff conversations, almost 50% of the sound peaks (noise above 80 dBA) in this study was attributed to human behavior in the form of staff conversation or television.

Sound elevations affect sleep among ICU patients, even ventilated patients. Using continuous 24-hour PSG with time-synchronized environmental monitoring, researchers studied seven ventilated patients in an ICU. They found that sound elevations occurred 36 plus or minus 20 (standard deviation) times per hour of sleep, and were responsible for 21 plus or minus 11% of total arousals and awakenings [63]. Using PSG monitoring and 80 dBA as a cut off, other researchers found similar results, with a very strong correlation ($r = 0.57$, $P = .0001$) between the number of sound peaks and arousals from sleep [64].

Patient care activities or interactions, such as mouth and eye care, wound care, bed bath, catheter care, and endotracheal suctioning, are another source of arousals or awakenings of patients. In a study of 60 patients in a surgical ICU, data were gathered for three consecutive nights. There was a mean of 51 patient interactions per patient per night, with the most frequent interactions occurring between 2 AM and 5 AM [65]. Another study of 50 patients from four different ICUs, with data from 147 nights, showed that the mean number of interactions was 43 per patient per night. A sleep promoting intervention was documented for only 1 of the 147 nights, and 62% of routine baths were provided between 11 PM and 6 AM [66].

Despite such dramatic numbers, some ICU patients manage to sleep, while others do not, but most have poor quality sleep. In a study of 22 medical ICU patients (20 were mechanically ventilated), using continuous PSG monitoring, all patients had sleep-wake cycle abnormalities and there were large variations in total sleep time [67]. Another study of 20 medical-surgical ICU patients (all were mechanically ventilated), showed the same results: that no patient had normal sleep patterns according to PSG [68]. Although in the former study, mean total sleep time was 8.8 plus or minus 5 hours per 24-hour period, and in the latter it was 7 plus or minus 2.5 hours per 24-hour period, these numbers should be viewed with caution. The standard deviation is quite wide, so some patients slept short times and others longer, and in both studies over 50% of electrophysiologic sleep was distributed throughout the daytime hours.

Although there are no well-controlled studies examining how sleep disturbance among ICU patients affects in-hospital outcomes, such as ICU or overall hospital length of stay, morbidity or mortality, one study evaluated patients' memories and experiences during their ICU stay, 6 months after they were discharged from the ICU. Of 1,433 patients admitted to the ICU, partly because of a mortality rate over 20%, only 464 patients completed the questionnaire. Although 73% of respondents described sleep as "good" or "good enough" during their ICU stay, 51% said they had dreams or nightmares during that time, of which 14% reported that those dreams or nightmares disturb their present day life. A total of 41% of patients reported general sleep disturbances at 6 months [69].

Sleep is dependent to some extent on light, the right kind, the right amount, and at the right time. This is a particular problem in critically ill patients, where continuous lighting and the absence of natural light are common and commonly accepted. Not only do these aspects of lighting negatively affect sleep, they have been implicated in the development of delirium [54]. For example, in a windowless critical care unit built in Great Britain in 1975, the percentage of patients experiencing delirium was twice the level noted in units with windows [70]. In a systematic review of patients' ICU experiences, impaired cognition occurred in 50% of the population in windowless units and in 41% of individuals in units with windows [71].

Artificial light from fluorescent bulbs can be harmful, and is associated with fatigue and headaches [72]. An often overlooked problem by doctors, nurses, and other staff who are younger than the average ICU patient, is that of glare [73]. This occurs when light is reflected off of surfaces such as glass, mirrors, shiny metal, and polished floors or surfaces. Young eyes can accommodate the glare, but older eyes have more difficulty doing so. Similarly, sudden exposure to any light, be it natural sun light or artificial lighting, can also blind or significantly impair vision of older persons.

Interventions

Nonpharmacologic interventions are preferable to the use of medication for sleep problems because of the risk associated with the use of sedating drugs in the elderly. These risks among hospitalized older persons include the risk of delirium, falls, hip fractures, dependency, and rebound insomnia [11–15]. No medication in this category is without some risk for an adverse drug event. Although newer agents continue to come to market, and are possibly safer if they have shorter half-lives and less abuse potential, caution is still advised. A good example of this was when zolpidem, a new generation of sleeping pills at the time, showed great promise. However, as Wang and colleagues [74] have shown, when new agents first become available, they appear to be safer than the "old" medications, but when studied in large populations, they still have hold potential risk for serious negative outcomes. Zolpidem use was associated with a significant increased risk of hip fracture (adjusted odds ratio or AOR 1.95; 95% CI, 1.09–3.51). Other psychotropic medication classes with significantly increased risks, included benzodiazepines (AOR 1.46; 95% CI, 1.21–1.76), antipsychotic medications (AOR 1.61; 95% CI, 1.29–2.01), and antidepressants (AOR 1.46; 95% CI, 1.22–1.75). For a more detailed description of pharmacologic approaches to insomnia in the elderly, especially related to safety profiles, other articles in this series of *The Clinics* are recommended.

Before describing some of the available evidence on protocols studied in sleep promotion, specific nonpharmacologic interventions to promote sleep, such as modifying the environment and interventions to promote relaxation and sleep, such as back massage and music therapy, are worth mentioning separately (Box 2).

One of the most modifiable sources of noise is staff conversation. In addition, turning down alarms, dimming the lights, rescheduling routine care, and being vigilant about blocking multidisciplinary care between midnight and 5 AM are recommended [75]. Another method of noise reduction is to post signs on the unit to remind staff and visitors to speak quietly. In many Chinese hospitals, signs reading "quiet please" are posted right above the nurses' stations and in the hallways of patient care areas [76]. Turning off equipment that is not being used and lowering volumes or alternatives to intercom use at night can help with environmental noise.

Backrubs or back massage techniques probably have the best available evidence for relaxation and sleep promotion. A technique called "slow-stroke back massage" has been traditionally used by nurses. Approximately 5 to 10 minutes of massage can induce a relaxation response, reduce the heart rate, respiratory rate, muscle tension, even decrease pain and anxiety, and improve sleep [77–79]. This type of back massage was used in the multicomponent study by McDowell and colleagues [80], which is discussed

---

Box 2. Check-list for evaluation of and interventions for insomnia among hospitalized older patients

H Herbal tea or warm milk
E Evaluate medication list for causes of insomnia
L Limit nighttime interruptions (eg, vital signs)
P Postpone morning labs
M Massage
E Evaluate daytime activity
S Sound reduction
L Light reduction at night
E Environment changes (eg, temperature of room, single room)
E Easy listening music or white sound
P Pain relief

below in more detail. Critical care patients receiving a 6-minute back massage versus routine nursing care experienced one additional hour of sleep per night in a study of cardiovascular ICU patients [81].

Music therapy was effective in reducing anxiety and pain, and in promoting relaxation among hospitalized patients in two studies [82,83]. Among cardiac surgical patients, improvement was seen in self-reported pain and sleep after receiving a postoperative music intervention [84]. According to White [83], the characteristics of music best suited for sleep and relaxation promotion are a tempo of approximately 60 beats per minute, composition of primarily low tones, and arrangement predominately by stringed instruments. The use of nonmusical tapes for relaxation has been studied. These typically involve sounds of the ocean or rain [85].

Although studies evaluating the use of aromatherapy for sleep promotion have not been as rigorous as the ones for massage or music, one study demonstrated that aromatherapy improved mood and decreased anxiety in a group of ICU patients [86]. In a special postoperative holistic care unit, nurses use 15-minute holistic interventions, such as essential oils, peppermint, and lavender, as part of their standard nursing practice [87].

Bright light pulses were studied in 10 patients with Alzheimer's disease on a research ward of a veteran's hospital. All patients had had sundowning behavior and sleep disturbances. After obtaining a week of baseline measurements, researchers exposed patients to 2 hours per day of bright light between 7 PM and 11 PM for 1 week. Clinical ratings of sleep-wakefulness on the evening nursing shift improved in eight of the ten patients. The proportion of total daily activity occurring during the nighttime decreased during the light-treatment week. More severe sundowning at baseline predicted greater clinical improvement [88].

Protocols

There are a limited number of published studies testing protocols which are based on the nonpharmacologic interventions above, but the ones which do exist are helpful in that they have demonstrated that protocols can be implemented. After review of the data, common implementation strategies will be reviewed.

McDowell and colleagues [80] studied the feasibility of and adherence to a three-part sleep protocol consisting of a back rub, a warm drink, and relaxation tapes. The nurses were instructed to offer the sleep protocol to any patient age 70 years or older who requested a sleep medication or complained of difficulty initiating sleep. If the patient refused, or the protocol was ineffective after 1 hour, the nurse proceeded with usual care. Usual care in this study was completely determined by the nurse, without any input from the researchers. The study enrolled 111 out of 175 (63%) eligible older hospitalized patients. Eligibility criteria were age greater than or equal to 70 years, admission during the study period, and ability to communicate in English.

Three important results came out of this study. First, overall adherence to the protocol, which was defined as doing at least one part of the three-part protocol, was 74%. This is quite acceptable, given that the researchers assessed the need for the protocol every day the subjects were in the study. Among the 111 subjects, the total number of days of "need" was 539 (for a mean of 4.9 plus or minus 5, standard deviation, days per patient). Of 539 days, subjects received at least part of the protocol on 400 days. Although only 9% received all three parts, 41% received two parts, and 24% received one part. Of the 26% of the time the protocol was not done, only 6% was nonadherence by nurses, and about 20% was because of subject refusal. Subjects refused the relaxation tapes most often (48% of the time), then warm drinks (39%), followed by massage (30%). The interventions were rarely medically contraindicated, 27 out of 539 subject days, for reasons such as strict supine position after a medical procedure, or nothing-by-mouth status or emesis.

The second important result was that the sleep protocol had a stronger association with quality of sleep than did patients who received a sedative or hypnotic drug through usual care.

The third finding, although not as strong because of the limitations of the study, was that the sleep protocol reduced the overall use of sedative hypnotic drugs on the study unit. The investigators found the rate of drug use in a baseline study group of comparable older subjects during 3 months before the introduction of the sleep protocol was 54% (51 out of 94), and only 31% (34 out of 111) during the intervention study [80].

To determine why this protocol was successful, one must look at the implementation of the protocol. As is so often seen in hospital and other health care systems, a good protocol is only as good as the implementation plan and follow through. For the McDowell study, there were at least five components necessary for success: (1) choosing protocol interventions that were relatively inexpensive (in terms of costs of equipment and nursing time); (2) easy access to the necessary equipment (the warm drinks, relaxation tapes, and massage information was kept in one designated are on one unit); (3) ongoing education sessions for the nursing staff (which started 2 months before the study, and occurred on all three nursing shifts on the unit); (4) written material for nurses, as well as for patients and families; and (5) reinforcement of the protocol with nurses, patients, and families by a geriatric clinical nurse.

In another nonrandomized study, called the "Sh-h-h-h Project," a multicomponent intervention was done. Certified nurse assistants (CNAs) completed an educational program about nonpharmacologic methods to promote sleep. One of the innovative tools used in this study were the "Sleep baskets," a midsize wicker basket with a list of possible interventions. This list served as a reminder for the CNAs, and gave subjects choices for sleep aides. Included on the list or in the basket were back rubs, warm drinks (milk or decaffeinated tea), aromatherapy (lavender to be placed on a tissue near the patient's pillow), warm blankets, relaxation music (the hospital's TV education channel offered 10 music and nature sound selections), "quiet" reminders and ear plugs, and closed doors reminders. Concerning the last part of the intervention, staff were reminded to use "quiet voices" after 10 PM and encouraged to avoid hallway conversations on the 11 PM to 7 AM shift. When possible, patients' doors were closed.

When a sleep basket was used, the night-shift CNAs recorded which interventions were used and the day-shift CNAs interviewed subjects. They asked the subjects to rate the quantity and quality of sleep and to identify which interventions were most helpful. Of 40 subjects, 15 (37.5%) subjects stated they slept "a lot"; 14 (35%) said, "a fair amount"; and 11 (27.5%) said "a little." When asked the general question of whether the interventions helped, 30 (75%) responded "yes." When asked if they felt rested on awakening, 32 (80%) responded "yes." The warm blankets were the most popular intervention (38 out of 40 subjects requested these), followed by the back rub (10 of 40 requests). All other interventions were requested by five or fewer subjects [89].

Although this study has some limitations (no report of which and how many subjects received pharmacologic interventions for sleep; how subjects were identified or screened for the interventions), its strengths are its feasibility and practicality. CNAs are the most likely members of the hospital health care team to identify insomnia among patients and may be the best first line in trying to help the patient before medications are requested.

Interventions to improve the ICU culture of noise as they relate to sleep disturbances have had modest success, but can be done. One group of investigators first identified which noises were amenable to behavior modification. Then they implemented their 3-week behavioral modification program on these results. They significantly reduced the 24-hour peak noise level and the mean peak noise level. They also decreased number of sound peaks that reached more than 79 dBA in all 6-hour blocks, except for the midnight to 6 AM time period [62]. Another study tried to affect noise levels by implementing simple nighttime guidelines in a surgical ICU. Although the study was successful in decreasing noise levels, peak noise levels, and number of acoustic identified alarms, overall noise levels were high both before and after implementation of the guidelines, and corresponded to a quiet office for noise level equivalents and to a busy restaurant for peak noise levels [90]. A surgical ICU was successful in decreasing noise intensity through implementation of a dedicated program of behavior change based on guidelines [55].

"Quiet-time" protocols and "nondisturbance" periods can be successful interventions. In one study, researchers directly observed 239 patients eight times each day before and after implementation of a protocol in which environmental sounds and lights were decreased during the 2 AM to 4 AM period and 2 PM to 4 PM period. The percentage of patients observed asleep was significantly higher during the months when the quiet-time period was implemented. The improved sleep was associated with decreased sound and light levels measured during the quiet-period intervention [91]. Another study introduced afternoon and nighttime nondisturbance periods. It showed reduced sleep disturbance factors (such as patient care interactions) and partly reduced noise levels. This study did not report on sleep outcomes [92].

In a study of 13 mechanically ventilated patients, who were being weaned from the ventilator, investigators randomly assigned subjects to either pressure support ventilation or proportional assist ventilation on the first night, and then crossed over to the alternative mode for the second night. Using PSG monitoring, arousals per hour of sleep time were higher when pressure support was used (mean 16, range 2–74) as compared with when proportional assist was used (mean 9, range 1–41). Overall sleep quality was significantly improved on the proportional assist ventilation mode [93].

Interventions, such as incorporation of windows or skylights in patient rooms or close by, may help [71]. The Society of Critical Care Medicine recommends that a maximum intensity of light used at night be 6.5 foot-candles for continuous lighting and 19 foot-candles for lighting used for short periods [94]. Some practical and logical interventions include use of indirect light, mounting of light fixtures behind the head of a patient's bed, and avoiding use of overhead procedure lights except when necessary [73]. The use of eye masks might be helpful in certain individuals who are accustomed to these, but they tend to create sensory deprivation and may increase risk of confusion [54]. Timing of light is as important as quality and quantity, as was seen in a study discussed above [90]. In this intervention trial to implement guidelines in a surgical ICU, although the result was a lower mean light disturbance intensity, this caused greater variability of light, which may also cause sleep disturbance.

Summary

Rates of insomnia and rates of use of sedative-hypnotic drugs among older hospitalized persons are high. Insomnia may represent undiagnosed sleep disorders or underlying medical or psychiatric problems. Evaluation and management of insomnia should target intrinsic (underlying medical illnesses, medications, or withdrawal from medications or alcohol) and extrinsic causes (hospital environment, patient care activities, noise, and medical technology or monitoring). Nonpharmacologic interventions are preferable, given the risks associated with sedating drugs (delirium, falls, hip fractures, dependency, and rebound insomnia). There is existing evidence to support the use of nonpharmacologic protocols. Implementation can be successful if the interventions are relatively inexpensive (in terms of costs of equipment and nursing time), use equipment that is practical and accessible, provide for ongoing staff education, include written material for nurses and patients, and regularly reinforce the sleep protocol.

References

[1] Bahr RT. Sleep-wake patterns in the aged. J Gerontol Nurs 1983;9:534–9.

[2] Black PH. Psychoneuroimmunology: brain and immunity. Science & Medicine 1995;2(6): 16–25.

[3] Spenceley SM. Sleep inquiry: a look with fresh eyes. Image J Nurs Sch 1993;25(3):249–56.

[4] Krachman SL, D'Alonzo GE, Criner GJ. Sleep in the intensive care unit. Chest 1995;107: 1713–20.

[5] Berlin RM. Management of insomnia in hospitalized patients. Ann Intern Med 1984;100(3): 398–404.

[6] Manabe K, Matsui T, Yamaya M, et al. Sleep patterns and mortality among elderly patients in a geriatric hospital. Gerontology 2000;46(6):318–22.

[7] Morrison D, Mayfield DG. Sleep insurance: a valid use of hypnotics? N C Med J 1972; 33(10):862–5.

[8] O'Reilly R, Rusnak C. The use of sedative-hypnotic drugs in a university teaching hospital. CMAJ 1990;142(6):585–9.

[9] Perry SW, Wu A. Rationale for the use of hypnotic agents in a general hospital. Ann Intern Med 1984;100(3):441–6.

[10] Zisselman MH, Rovner BW, Yuen EJ, et al. Sedative-hypnotic use and increased hospital stay and costs in older people. J Am Geriatr Soc 1996;44(11):1371–4.

[11] Bowen JD, Larson EB. Drug-induced cognitive impairment. Defining the problem and finding solutions. Drugs Aging 1993;3(4):349–57.

[12] Gottlieb GL. Sleep disorders and their management. Special considerations in the elderly. Am J Med 1990;88(3A):29S–33S.

[13] Campbell AJ. Drug treatment as a cause of falls in old age. A review of the offending agents. Drugs Aging 1991;1(4):289–302.

[14] Foy A, O'Connell D, Henry D, et al. Benzodiazepine use as a cause of cognitive impairment in elderly hospital inpatients. J Gerontol A Biol Sci Med Sci 1995;50(2):M99–106.

[15] Grad RM. Benzodiazepines for insomnia in community-dwelling elderly: a review of benefit and risk. J Fam Pract 1995;41(5):473–81.

[16] Joshi S. Current concepts in the management of delirium. Mo Med 2007;104(1):58–62.

[17] King KB, Parinello KA. Patient perceptions of recovery from coronary artery bypass grafting after discharge from the hospital. Heart Lung 1988;17:708–15.

[18] Tack BB, Gillis CL. Nurse-monitored cardiac recovery: a description of the first 8 weeks. Heart Lung 1990;19:491–9.

[19] Redeker NS. Symptoms reported by older and middle-aged adults after coronary bypass surgery. Clin Nurs Res 1993;2:148–59.

[20] Schaefer KM, Swavely D, Rothenberger C, et al. Sleep disturbances post coronary artery bypass surgery. Prog Cardiovasc Nurs 1996;11:5–14.

[21] Meissner HH, Riemer A, Santiago SM, et al. Failure of physician documentation of sleep complaints in hospitalized patients. West J Med 1998;169(3):146–9.

[22] Ancoli-Israel S. Epidemiology of sleep disorders. Clin Geriatr Med 1989;5(2):347–62.

[23] American Psychiatric Association. Diagnostic and statistical manual of mental disorders: DSM-IV. 4th edition. Washington (DC): American Psychiatric Publishing; 1994.

[24] Francis J, Martin D, Kapoor WN. A prospective study of delirium in hospitalized elderly. JAMA 1990;263:1097–101.

[25] Inouye SK, Viscoli CM, Horwitz RI, et al. A predictive model for delirium in hospitalized elderly medical patients based on admission characteristics. Ann Intern Med 1993;19: 474–81.

[26] Johnson JC, Gottlieb GL, Sullivan E, et al. Using DSM-III criteria to diagnose delirium in elderly general medical patients. J Gerontol A Biol Sci Med Sci 1990;45:M113–9.

[27] Ely EW, Shintani A, Truman B, et al. Delirium as a predictor of mortality in mechanically ventilated patients in the intensive care unit. JAMA 2004;291:1753–62.

[28] Dyer CB, Ashton CM, Teasdale TA. Postoperative delirium. A review of 80 primary data-collection studies. Arch Intern Med 1995;155:461–5.

[29] Inouye SK. Delirium in hospitalized older patients: recognition and risk factors. J Geriatr Psychiatry Neurol 1998;11:118–25.

[30] Lyons WL. Delirium in postacute and long-term care. J Am Med Dir Assoc 2006;7(4): 254–61.

[31] Miller DK, Lewis LM, Nork MJ, et al. Controlled trial of a geriatric case-finding and liaison service in an emergency department. J Am Geriatr Soc 1996;44(5):513–20.

[32] Inouye SK, Foreman MD, Mion LC, et al. Nurses' recognition of delirium and its symptoms: comparison of nurse and researcher ratings. Arch Intern Med 2001;161:2467–73.

[33] Lyness JM. Delirium: masquerades and misdiagnosis in elderly inpatients. J Am Geriatr Soc 1990;38:1235–8.

[34] Pompei P, Foreman M, Rudberg MA, et al. Delirium in hospitalized older persons: outcomes and predictors. J Am Geriatr Soc 1994;42:809–15.

[35] Cole M, McCusker J, Dendukuri N, et al. The prognostic significance of subsyndromal delirium in elderly medical inpatients. J Am Geriatr Soc 2003;51:754–60.

[36] McCusker J, Kakuma R, Abrahamowicz M. Predictors of functional decline in hospitalized elderly patients: a systematic review. J Gerontol A Biol Sci Med Sci 2002;57:M569–77.

[37] McCusker J, Cole M, Abrahamowicz M. Environmental risk factors for delirium in hospitalized older people. J Am Geriatr Soc 2001;49:1327–34.

[38] McCusker J, Cole M, Dendukuri N, et al. The course of delirium in older medical inpatients: a prospective study. J Gen Intern Med 2003;18:696–704.

[39] Rockwood K. Educational interventions in delirium. Dement Geriatr Cogn Disord 1999;10: 426–9.

[40] Inouye SK, Rushing JT, Foreman MD, et al. Does delirium contribute to poor hospital outcomes? a three-site epidemiologic study. J Gen Intern Med 1998;13:234–42.

[41] O'Keeffe S, Lavan J. The prognostic significance of delirium in older hospital patients. J Am Geriatr Soc 1997;45:174–8.

[42] Thomas RI, Cameron DJ, Fahs MC. A prospective study of delirium and prolonged hospital stay. Exploratory study. Arch Gen Psychiatry 1998;45:937–40.

[43] Vitiello MV. Effective treatments for age-related sleep disturbances. Geriatrics 1999;54(11): 47–52.

[44] Rocha FL, Hara C, Rodrigues CV, et al. Is insomnia a marker for psychiatric disorders in general hospitals? Sleep Med 2005;6(6):549–53.

[45] Bliwise DL. Sleep in normal aging and dementia. Sleep 1993;16(1):40–81.

[46] Flaherty JH. "Who's taking your 5th vital sign?". J Gerontol A Biol Sci Med Sci 2001;56(7): M397–9.

[47] Flaherty JH, Rudolph J, Shay K, et al. Delirium is a serious and under-recognized problem: Why assessment of mental status should be the 6th vital sign. J Am Med Dir Assoc 2007;8(6):273–5.

[48] Vitiello MV, Bliwise DL, Prinz PN. Sleep in Alzheimer's disease and the sundown syndrome. Neurology 1992;42(7 Suppl 6):83–93.

[49] Ancoli-Israel S. Sleep problems in older adults: putting myths to bed. Geriatrics 1997;52(1): 20–30.

[50] Lenhart SE, Buysse DJ. Treatment of insomnia in hospitalized patients. Ann Pharmacother 2001;35(11):1449–57.

[51] Wetterling T, Kanitz RD, Besters B, et al. A new rating scale for the assessment of the alcohol-withdrawal syndrome (AWS scale). Alcohol Alcohol 1997;32(6):753–60.

[52] Shaw JM, Kolesar GS, Sellers EM, et al. Development of optimal treatment tactics for alcohol withdrawal. I. Assessment and effectiveness of supportive care. J Clin Psychopharmacol 1981;1(6):382–7.

[53] Vinall PE. Design technology: what you need to know about circadian rhythms in healthcare design. J Health Care Inter Des 1997;9:141–4.

[54] Fontaine DK, Briggs LP, Pope-Smith B. Designing humanistic critical care environments. Crit Care Nurs Q 2001;24(3):21–34.

[55] Moore MM, Nguyen D, Nolan SP, et al. Interventions to reduce decibel levels on patient care units. Am Surg 1998;64:894–9.

[56] Tullman DF, Dracup K. Creating a healing environment for elders. AACN Clinical Issues Advanced Practice in Acute and Critical Care 2000;11:34–50.

[57] Christensen M. Noise levels in a general surgical ward: a descriptive study. J Clin Nurs 2005; 14(2):156–64.

[58] Urbankova J, Quiroz R, Kucher N, et al. Intermittent pneumatic compression and deep vein thrombosis prevention. A meta-analysis in postoperative patients. Thromb Haemost 2005; 94(6):1181–5.

[59] Mazzone C, Chiodo GF, Sandercock P, Miccio M, Salvi R. Physical methods for preventing deep vein thrombosis in stroke. Cochrane Database of Systematic Reviews 2004;(4):CD001922.

[60] Romano M. Personal space. Guidelines call for only private rooms. Mod Healthc 2005; 35(31):20.

[61] Romano M. Going solo. Private-rooms-only provision for new hospital construction stirs controversy. Mod Healthc 2004;34(48):36, 38.

[62] Kahn DM, Cook TE, Carlisle CC, et al. Identification and modification of environmental noise in an ICU setting. Chest 1998;114(2):535–40.

[63] Gabor JY, Cooper AB, Crombach SA, et al. Contribution of the intensive care unit environment to sleep disruption in mechanically ventilated patients and healthy subjects. Am J Respir Crit Care Med 2003;167(5):708–15.

[64] Aaron JN, Carlisle CC, Carskadon MA, et al. Environmental noise as a cause of sleep disruption in an intermediate respiratory care unit. Sleep 1996;19(9):707–10.

[65] Celik S, Oztekin D, Akyolcu N, et al. Sleep disturbance: the patient care activities applied at the night shift in the intensive care unit. J Clin Nurs 2005;14(1):102–6.

[66] Tamburri LM, DiBrienza R, Zozula R, et al. Nocturnal care interactions with patients in critical care units. Am J Crit Care 2004;13(2):102–12.

[67] Freedman NS, Gazendam J, Levan L, et al. Abnormal sleep/wake cycles and the effect of environmental noise on sleep disruption in the intensive care unit. Am J Respir Crit Care Med 2001;163(2):451–7.

[68] Cooper AB, Thornley KS, Young GB, et al. Sleep in critically ill patients requiring mechanical ventilation. Chest 2000;117:809–18.

[69] Granja C, Lopes A, Moreira S, et al. JMIP Study Group. Patients' recollections of experiences in the intensive care unit may affect their quality of life. Crit care 2005;9(2):R96–109.

[70] Duffy TM, Florell JM. Intensive care units. J Health Care Inter Des 1990;2:167–79.

[71] Stein-Parbury J, McKinley S. Patients' experiences of being in an intensive care unit: a select literature review. Am J Crit Care 2000;9:20–7.

[72] Fontaine DK. Measurement of nocturnal sleep patterns in trauma patients. Heart Lung 1989;18:402–10.

[73] Williams MA. Physical environment of the intensive care unit and elderly patients. Crit Care Nurs Q 1989;12(1):52–60.

[74] Wang PS, Bohn RL, Glynn RJ, et al. Zolpidem use and hip fractures in older people. J Am Geriatr Soc 2001;49(12):1685–90.

[75] Edwards GB, Schuring LM. Sleep protocol: a research-based practice change. Crit Care Nurse 1993;13(2):84–8.

[76] Flaherty JH, Liu ML, Ding L, et al. China: The aging giant. J Am Geriatr Soc 2007;55: 1295–300.

[77] Fakouri C, Jones P. Relaxation Rx: slow stroke back rub. J Gerontol Nurs 1987;13(2):32–5.

[78] Ferrell-Torry AT, Glick OJ. The use of therapeutic massage as a nursing intervention to modify anxiety and the perception of cancer pain. Cancer Nurs 1993;16(2):93–101.

[79] Labyak SE, Metzger BL. The effects of effleurage backrub on the physiological components of relaxation: A meta-analysis. Nurs Res 1997;46:59–62.

[80] McDowell JA, Mion LC, Lydon TJ, et al. A nonpharmacologic sleep protocol for hospitalized older patients. J Am Geriatr Soc 1998;46(6):700–5.

[81] Richards KC. Effect of a back massage and relaxation intervention on sleep in critically ill patients. Am J Crit Care 1998;7:288–99.

[82] Byers JF, Smyth KA. Effect of a music intervention on noise annoyance, heart rate, and blood pressure in cardiac surgery patients. Am J Crit Care 1997;6(3):183–91.

[83] White JM. Effects of relaxing music on cardiac autonomic balance and anxiety after acute myocardial infarction. Am J Crit Care 1999;8(4):220–30.

[84] Zimmerman L, Nieveen J, Barnason S, et al. The effects of music interventions on postoperative pain and sleep in coronary artery bypass graft (CABG) patients. Sch Inq Nurs Pract 1996;10(2):153–70.

[85] Williamson JW. The effects of ocean sounds on sleep after coronary artery bypass graft surgery. Am J Crit Care 1992;1(1):91–7.

[86] Dunn C, Sleep J, Collet D. Sensing an improvement: An experimental study to evaluate the use of aroma therapy, massage, and periods of rest in intensive care units. J Adv Nurs 1995; 21:34–40.

[87] Horrigan B. Region's hospital opens holistic nursing unit. Alt Ther 2000;6(4):92–3.

[88] Satlin A, Volicer L, Ross V, et al. Bright light treatment of behavioral and sleep disturbances in patients with Alzheimer's disease. Am J Psychiatry 1992;149(8):1028–32.

[89] Robinson SB, Weitzel T, Henderson L. The Sh-h-h-h project. Nonpharmacological interventions. Holist Nurs Pract 2005;19(6):263–6.

[90] Walder B, Francioli D, Meyer JJ, et al. Effects of guidelines implementation in a surgical intensive care unit to control nighttime light and noise levels. Crit Care Med 2000;28(7): 2242–7.

[91] Olson DM, Borel CO, Laskowitz DT, et al. Quiet time: a nursing intervention to promote sleep in neurocritical care units. Am J Crit Care 2001;10(2):74–8.

[92] Monsen MG, Edell-Gustafsson UM. Noise and sleep disturbance factors before and after implementation of a behavioural modification programme. Intensive Crit Care Nurs 2005; 21(4):208–19.

[93] Bosma K, Ferreyra G, Ambrogio C, et al. Patient-ventilator interaction and sleep in mechanically ventilated patients: pressure support versus proportional assist ventilation. Crit Care Med 2007;35(4):1048–54.

[94] Guidelines/Practice Parameters Committee of the American College of Critical Care Medicine, Society of critical care medicine. Guidelines for intensive care unit design. Crit Care Med 1995;23:582–8.

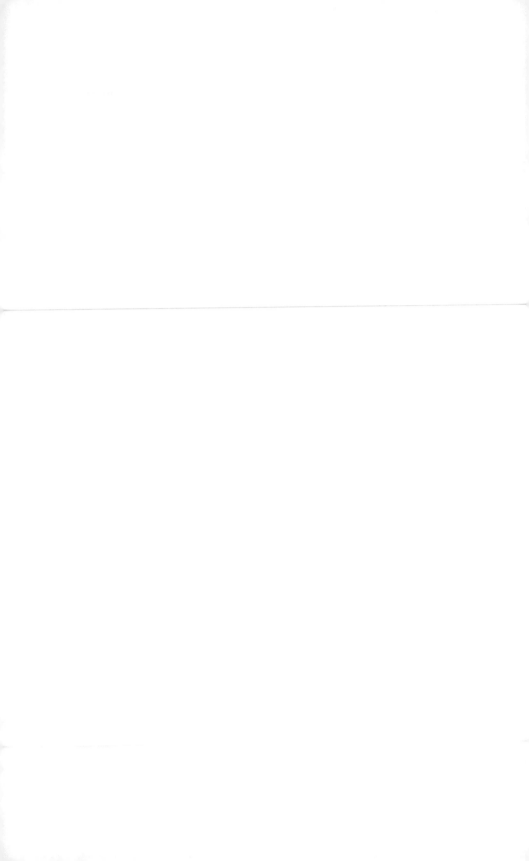

ELSEVIER
SAUNDERS

CLINICS IN
GERIATRIC
MEDICINE

Clin Geriatr Med 24 (2008) 69–81

The Demented Elder with Insomnia

Miguel A. Paniagua, MD[a],*,
Elizabeth W. Paniagua, MD[b]

[a]Division of Gerontology & Geriatric Medicine, Saint Louis University School of Medicine,
1402 South Grand Boulevard, Room M238, Saint Louis, MO 63104, USA
[b]Saint Louis, MO, USA

The paucity of research in the area of sleep disturbance in elder individuals is no more promising in the demented elder population. Nevertheless, insomnia is neither a normal part of aging nor an accepted consequence of dementia; however, the severity of the disordered sleep and daytime napping tend to parallel that of the dementia as it progresses (Table 1) [1]. Nighttime behavioral abnormalities and sleep disturbance affect up to one half of all dementia patients and run the gamut of severity.

Physiology

The loss or damage of neuronal pathways in the suprachiasmatic nucleus, the area that initiates and maintains sleep as well as changes in the circadian rhythm, likely contributes to sleep disturbances in elders with dementia. A discussion of polysomnographic findings in older adults is discussed elsewhere in this edition of *The Clinics*. In Alzheimer's disease (AD) patients, as opposed to elder controls, loss of cholinergic neurons in the nucleus basalis and numerous other sites, is likely responsible for a decrease in rapid eye movement (REM) sleep noted on polysomnography of AD patients. Other notable, but less specific changes in AD patients, include increased sleep fragmentation and arousals, increase in stage 1 (light) sleep, decrease in total sleep time, and decreased sleep spindles and K complexes [2,3]. Poor quality nighttime sleep increases daytime sleepiness and napping, thereby leading to poor sleep hygiene and insomnia. Melatonin levels have also been reported to be significantly lower in AD patients than elderly controls, and the rhythm may be dampened or temporally disturbed [4].

* Corresponding author.
E-mail address: mpaniag1@slu.edu (M.A. Paniagua).

0749-0690/08/$ - see front matter © 2008 Elsevier Inc. All rights reserved.
doi:10.1016/j.cger.2007.08.010   *geriatric.theclinics.com*

Table 1
Characteristic sleep changes in dementia

Sleep characteristic	Resultant effect
Disruptive sleep pattern on EEG	Increases with dementia severity
Wakefulness after sleep onset	
Nighttime awakenings	
Nighttime wandering	
Daytime napping	
Latency to first rapid eye movement sleep episode	
Stage 1 sleep	
Sundowning	
Total sleep time (TST)	Decrease with dementia severity
Sleep efficiency	
Rapid eye movement sleep	
Stage 3 sleep	
Stage 4 sleep	

Impact of sleep impairment in demented elders

The impact of sleep impairment in dementia patients and their caregivers can be profound. The effect on caregivers, who are awakened by the affected patient, is a prominent and disturbing phenomenon that often leads to institutionalization of the elder [4–8]. Additionally, declining physical and psychologic health status among caregivers has been shown to adversely affect the health of the demented elder with insomnia.

The cognitive effects of insomnia are many, and are compounded in delirious elders who have a compromised cognitive reserve at baseline. It stands to reason that insomnia often plays a role in both the etiology and the presentation of delirium in some cases. Loss of sleep can have a variety of physical consequences for a demented elder and their caregivers. The insomnia and resultant treatment attempts are equally implicated in the potential sequelae, ranging from excessive daytime somnolence to falls, accidents, and injuries. Insomnia can lead to other adverse effects in the older patient, and may lead to a nearly two-fold increase in 2-year mortality [9].

Functional sequelae of insomnia in dementia patients

It has been widely reported in the literature that sedative-hypnotic medication use predisposes the older patient to falls. However, the majority of studies do not consider the possibility that sleep deprivation or insomnia in and of itself may contribute to falls [10]. Additionally, cognitive deficits may worsen in the face of untreated insomnia, thereby making management of the underlying dementia more challenging [11].

Risk factors for poor sleep in dementia

Insomnia, sleep-disordered breathing, and anxiety are more prevalent in elders with dementia and other neurodegenerative disorders than elders without such neurologic disorders. Behavioral, antianxiety, and antidepressant treatments have been shown to help nighttime awakenings in these patients [12]. Overall, elderly patients with underlying dementia or cognitive impairment are more prone to developing delirium. Similarly, up to 60% of nursing home residents, many of whom have some degree of cognitive impairment, have delirium [13].

Institutionalization increases the risk of sleep disruption through a combination of underlying physiologic abnormalities (such as incontinence and nocturia) and external environmental factors (such as sleep interruption by staff and poor lighting). These factors may adversely affect circadian rhythms. Institutionalized elders are exposed to less bright light and daytime physical activity. They also have more nighttime light exposure that may suppress melatonin and increase nocturnal wakefulness [14].

Medications commonly used to treat behavioral disturbances in the demented elder also have adverse effects on the sleep-wake cycle (Table 2) [15–21]. Research also suggests a genetic contributor to poor sleep in some demented patients. In one study, AD patients showed an increased likelihood of sleep disturbance with a genetic polymorphism of the monoamine oxidase A enzyme [22].

Diagnosis and evaluation

Clinical presentation

The clinical presentation of sleep disturbance in Alzheimer's disease is variable and, to some extent, subject to the perception of the affected caregiver and the patient with dementia. What constitutes a disturbance in sleep can range from agitation or sundowning to wandering or sleep disordered breathing. Caregivers may report more than one sleep complaint, as these symptoms often coexist in the same individual. Symptoms may or may not be distressing to the patient, depending in part upon the severity of the dementia.

Evaluation

The evaluation of insomnia in the demented elder should first begin with an assessment of potential underlying causes. This includes a complete medical, psychiatric, and sleep assessment, including review of recent medication use and timing of doses. If available, patient or caregiver reports (or diary) of sleep for the preceding 1 to 2 weeks can be useful in determining a pattern of sleep disruption that includes the onset, duration, total sleep time, frequency, and severity of insomnia symptoms. Consideration of the elder's

Table 2
Frequently used medications with adverse effects on sleep in demented elders

Medication class	Comment
Laxatives	Increased frequency of defecation
Antihypertensives	Diuretics
	Can cause nocturia
	Beta-blocker
	May slightly decrease total sleep time (limited data)
	May affect mood
	May impair melatonin secretion (uncertain clinical significance) [19,20]
	Clonidine
	May cause drowsiness
	Dose-related reduction in quantity of REM sleep
Psychotropics	Antidepressants
	SSRIs may decrease REM sleep
	Alcohol
	Limited data in elderly
	May reduce sleep efficiency, REM sleep and total sleep time
	Even hours after consumption [17]
Analgesics	Codeine
	May have anticholinergic effects
	Untreated pain may contribute to sleep difficulties
Cholinesterase Inhibitors	Increased REM sleep
	Possible bothersome and vivid dreams
Sympathomimetics and Stimulants	Decongestants
	Many agents with varying effects
	Combination products may contain anticholinergic agents
	Nicotine
	Cigarettes associated with prolonged sleep latency and decreased total sleep time [21]
	Nicotine patch may promote vivid dreams
	Increased sleep fragmentation [18]
	Caffeine
	Decreases sleep propensity even at low levels
Bronchodilators	Varying effects
	May cause increased alertness
	Sleep may be enhanced by improvement in respiratory difficulties
Endocrinologic agents	Corticosteroids
	May cause increased alertness
	Potential for dosing/timing related effects
	Progesterone
	Possible hypnotic effect
	Respiratory stimulant
Anti-Parkinsonian drugs	Levodopa
	Increased daytime sleepiness
	Severe and possibly dose-related effects [16].
Antiepileptics	Phenytoin
	Drowsiness
	Can reduce REM sleep
	Sleep disruption
	Gabapentin
	May improve sleep through fewer awakenings [15]

Abbreviations: REM, rapid eye movement; SSRI, selective serotonin reuptake inhibitor.

living environment (whether home, a recent change, or in an institutional setting) should also be evaluated for potential extrinsic contributors to insomnia. Furthermore, determining the patient's sleep hygiene practices, diet, alcohol intake, and smoking history could provide clues to other common contributors to the sleep disruption. In the case of demented elders, the role of caregivers and family in providing collateral information cannot be stressed enough, particularly in the institutional setting.

Generally speaking, as is the case in all geriatric syndromes, it is uncommon to find a single precipitating cause of one's insomnia. Likely, interplay between underlying medical illnesses and their treatments, sleep hygiene, and environment are all contributing to the problem. For this reason, establishing the diagnosis becomes a clinical challenge. Primary sleep disorders (such as sleep disordered breathing, restless legs syndrome, and periodic limb movement disorder) are more common with aging and the clinical identification of these becomes more difficult in demented elders. Great care should be taken in considering these disorders, as they can potentially exacerbate or contribute to cognitive impairment syndromes and sundowning.

Although tools, such as the nighttime behavior scale of the Neuropsychiatric Inventory [23], the Epworth Sleepiness Scale [24], and the Pittsburgh Sleep Quality Inventory [25,26] have been used in studies of this population, there is no single screening instrument for the demented elder with insomnia universally used in clinical practice. Kamel and Gammack have outlined an approach to the elder patient with insomnia, which has been adapted for use in the demented elder (Box 1) [27].

Sundowning

Sundowning is a poorly understood phenomenon. It is defined as a worsening in behavioral symptoms, as described by caregivers, that occurs mostly in the afternoon and evening in individuals with dementia. Sundowning is likely caused by disruption to circadian rhythms as dementia progresses [28]. Sundowning, in contrast to general agitation during other times of the day or night, correlates highly with rates of cognitive decline in affected patients [29]. Sundowning behavior in Alzheimer's patients is also associated with an increased rate of caregiver stress.

Sleep disordered breathing

The prevalence of sleep disordered breathing (SDB) is higher in older adults in general, and even more so in demented elders. Most of these cases involve obstructive sleep apnea [30]. SDB is associated with agitated behaviors in demented elders and can be more severe. Treatment of SDB, as an underlying cause of insomnia, can decrease agitation and thereby ease caregiver burden in those who remain community-dwelling [31]. A more extensive discussion of sleep-disordered breathing is included elsewhere in *The Clinics*.

Box 1. Approach to the demented elder with insomnia

Sleep History
Obtain from patient, caregivers, staff and family
Confirm the presence of insomnia
Identify the symptom (onset, duration, pattern, and severity)
Evaluate 24-hour sleep/wakefulness patterns
Review 1- to 2-week caregiver sleep diary or nursing notes
Evaluate the personal, institutional, and societal impact of the
  sleep disorder

Identify Causes and Contributing Risk Factors
Primary sleep disorders
Medical illness
Psychiatric illness
Behavioral
Environmental (particularly in case of hospital or institutional
  setting)
Medications

Evaluation and Management
Comprehensive physical exam
Targeted laboratory studies
Discuss the expectations with patient, caregivers, family and staff
Initiate effective treatment of primary etiology (if applicable)
Sleep hygiene measures
Nonpharmacologic measures
Pharmacologic intervention (as a last resort)
Referral to sleep specialist if necessary

Treatment

Considerations before selecting treatment

Before choosing a treatment strategy for insomnia in a demented patient, all possible diagnostic and coexisting or exacerbating conditions should be considered and addressed. In frail demented elders, symptom reporting or signs of illness can be subtle or all together absent. For these reasons, the presence of a secondary cause of insomnia should always be considered. For example, acute delirium because of an underlying illness can have insomnia as a feature of the initial presentation. A hallmark sign of untreated or under-treated depression can also be nighttime agitation or insomnia. Similarly, untreated or under-treated pain or pain syndromes can predictably lead to poor sleep. Polypharmacy, including a change in medication regimen that temporally relates to the insomnia, may lead to crucial clues in the etiology. It therefore stands to reason that the first-line therapeutic strategy for insomnia in the demented elder should be directed at improving sleep hygiene [27].

Challenges in treatment of insomnia in the demented elder

Treatment of insomnia in the geriatric patient is challenging to begin with, and is compounded when considering the patient with dementia. At baseline, demented elders present with a spectrum of memory problems and states of consciousness that can make them resistant or intolerant of treatment regimens. The use of interventions, such as continuous positive airway pressure (CPAP) for obstructive sleep apnea, a prevalent disease in the elder population, can be problematic in demented adults. With proper reassurance and supportive care, CPAP can generally be tolerated by individuals with mild to moderate dementia.

Cholinesterase inhibitors are the mainstay of treatment for dementia Alzheimer's type, but their use has been associated with increased insomnia, sleep disruption, and even vivid dreams. Sleep tends to be less affected with use of rivastigmine and galantamine, as opposed to donepezil [4].

As dementia progresses, so does the likelihood that an institutional setting, such as assisted living or nursing home, will be necessary. With institutionalization, environmental barriers to proper and normalized sleep become more likely. Furthermore, demented elders have less neurophysiologic reserve to tolerate disruptions in equilibrium. This enhances their sensitivity to the sedating properties of medications (especially psychoactives), the intended mechanism of action of sleep medications.

Nonpharmacologic

Light therapy

Like other treatments for insomnia in demented elders, particularly those who are institutionalized, intensive light therapy has also been sporadically studied. Bright light therapy used during wake hours, particularly if simulating dawn and dusk, can reduce agitation and improve sleep and circadian rhythms in elders with dementia [32,33]. In reality, it is often difficult to reliably expose demented elders in the institutional setting to regular natural or intensive light, especially when patient mobility is limited and facility staffing is inadequate. The optimal light frequency and light dose required for best possible effects in this population is not yet known.

Behavioral management and sleep hygiene

Implementation of proper sleep habits and routines, either in the home or institutional setting, are key to ensuring restful and restorative sleep in demented elders (Box 2). The nighttime insomnia treatment and education for Alzheimer's disease study examined whether behavioral interventions

Box 2. Behavioral strategies for improving sleep in persons with dementia

Sleep-wake practices
- Maintain a consistent bed and rising time
- Develop a relaxing, quiet bedtime routine
- Limit daytime napping to a short period in the morning or early afternoon

Environmental guidelines
- Spend time out of doors during the daytime in natural light
- Keep in-home living areas as brightly lit as possible during the day
- Keep sleeping areas dark at night and do not watch TV after the lights are out
- Use nightlights to avoid using overhead bright lights when getting up at night
- Make sure lights in bathrooms, halls, smoke detectors, and streetlights do not shine in your eyes while in bed
- Reduce household, outside traffic, and neighborhood noise in sleeping areas
- Ensure sleeping areas are a comfortable temperature; avoid overheating
- Keep pets away from sleeping areas at night
- If bed partners are disrupting sleep, consider whether separate beds, mattresses, or bedrooms might be helpful

Dietary and health guidelines
- Restrict use of caffeine (including chocolate), alcohol, and tobacco, particularly in the evening
- Establish regular meal times; avoid heavy or rich food late in the evening
- If hungry, a light bedtime snack can reduce nighttime awakenings that are caused by hunger
- Avoid excessive evening fluid intake and empty the bladder before going to bed
- Be aware that many prescription or over-the-counter medications can adversely affect sleep
- Talk with your physician about strategies to reduce musculoskeletal pain if it is contributing to nighttime awakenings
- Exercise regularly and moderately; avoid stimulating exercise after dinnertime

From McCurry SM, Logsdon RG, Vitiello MV, et al. Treatment of sleep and nighttime disturbances in Alzheimer's disease: a behavior management approach. Sleep Medicine 2004;5:373–7; with permission.

could improve sleep in community-dwelling AD patients. The focus of the intervention was sleep education for caregivers on good sleep practices, behavior management, increased daytime activity, and light exposure in demented elders. Although a small sample size, the study showed that demented patients with sleep problems have the potential to benefit from behavioral techniques, such as sleep hygiene education, daily exercise or walking, and increased light exposure [12,34–36].

Additionally, proper sleep hygiene also includes abstinence from substances that may adversely affect sleep in the demented elder. Alcohol may be used to self-medicate for insomnia, and when used as a hypnotic can decrease sleep latency, decrease REM sleep, and cause rebound insomnia. Frequent arousals during the night, either because of increased nocturia or spontaneous, are also present. These arousals are common with use of sympathomimetics and stimulants, such as nicotine and caffeine. Caffeine can also increase sleep latency and decrease efficiency of sleep. These effects are compounded by the slowed metabolism and smaller volume of distribution of these substances with aging.

Pharmacologic

Despite an ever-growing body of literature on both insomnia and behavioral disturbance in demented elders, there is no clear standard-of-care in the pharmacologic treatment of insomnia in this population. Further guideline development and research is needed in the areas of drug alternatives and safe prescribing [37–39]. Pharmacologic treatment of the demented elder with insomnia should be reserved for those deemed to have primary insomnia and who have not responded to more conservative, nonpharmacologic interventions. If the decision is made to treat with medication, the lowest possible effective dose should be used for a time-limited trial, and "as needed" dosing should be the rule, as opposed to scheduled doses (such as two to four times per week only for no more than 3–4 weeks, if possible).

Prescribed treatments should continue to be used in concert with nonpharmacologic and sleep hygiene measures. Use of these medications should be tapered or discontinued gradually, mindful of potential for rebound insomnia after discontinuation. The signs and symptoms of rebound insomnia can be subtle but can also manifest with overt agitation or disorientation in the demented elder. Pharmacotherapy for this population requires due diligence on the part of the clinician. Further information on specific pharmacologic agents is described in detail elsewhere in this issue.

When faced with a severely agitated individual with nighttime sleep disruption, antipsychotic therapy is frequently considered. The Agency for Health care Research and Quality's summary on the off-label use of atypical antipsychotics states that there is some medium-level evidence for the use of quetiapine, olanzapine, and risperidone in reducing agitation and behavioral disturbances in elders with dementia, which may secondarily improve sleep

Table 3
Sleep-associated side effects of atypical antipsychotics in demented elders

Side Effects	Olanzapine	Risperidone	Aripiprazole	Quetiapine	Ziprasidone
Extrapyramidal symptoms (uncontrollable movements)	▬▬	▬	▬	INSF	▬
Agitation	INSF	INSF	▬▬▬	INSF	INSF
Gait disturbance	▬	▬	INSF	INSF	INSF
Fatigue	▬	▬	▬▬	INSF	INSF
Sleepiness	▬▬▬	▬▬▬	▬▬▬	▬▬▬▬▬	▬
Pain	INSF	INSF	▬▬▬▬▬	INSF	INSF
Gastrointestinal symptoms	INSF	☐	▬▬▬	▬	INSF
Urinary symptoms	▬	■	▬▬▬▬▬	INSF	INSF

The length of the bar indicates how many people typically experience the harmful effect.	
▬▬▬▬▬	21-50%
▬▬▬	11-20%
▬	5-10%
■	Less than 5%
☐	The harmful side effect occurred more often in people taking placebo (inactive substance) than in people taking the drug.
INSF	Insufficient evidence.

Adapted from Saha S, Robinson S, Bianco T, et al. Efficacy and comparative effectiveness of off-label use of atypical antipsychotics. Portland (OR): The Southern California/RAND Evidence-based Practice Center, The Agency for Healthcare Research and Quality (AHRQ). The John M. Eisenberg Center; 2007; with permission.

in these individuals. Conversely, some side effects of these medications may not directly improve sleep but can indirectly worsen sleep. These include dry mouth, peripheral edema, and gastrointestinal or urinary symptoms resulting in constipation, frequent waking, and increased toileting. These side effects may be less prevalent in those taking aripiprazole, and more so with olanzapine and risperidone. Side effect profile should be considered before selecting an appropriate agent (Table 3). The greatest concern with the use of atypical antipsychotics continues to be the association with increased risk of stroke (specifically risperidone and olanzapine) and death in elders with dementia. These medications should be used with caution in those with vascular risk factors, as there is little data on longer-term side effects [40].

Melatonin

Melatonin is a pineal hormone whose secretion is stimulated by dark conditions and inhibited by light. The secretion of melatonin decreases with advancing age. Currently, there is no standardization or regulation of available preparations of this supplement, and few randomized controlled trials have been performed in demented elders. Although an absence of any significant adverse effects was seen among the demented individuals, the magnitude of effect in studies was minimal at best [41].

Summary

Insomnia in demented elders is a challenge to clinicians and caregivers alike. The evaluation should focus on easily remedied sources of sleep disturbance, such as medications, environmental factors, or contributing medical conditions. One should always consider the possibility of a primary sleep disorder when evaluating demented elders with sleep disturbance. Demented elders are no less worthy of targeted interventions than their cognitively-intact counterparts, provided one is mindful of their relative sensitivity to both pharmacologic and many of the recommended nonpharmacologic interventions.

References

[1] Grace JB, Walker MP, McKeith IG. A comparison of sleep profiles in patients with dementia with lewy bodies and Alzheimer's disease. Int J Geriatr Psychiatry 2000;15(11):1028–33.
[2] Avidan AY. Sleep and neurologic problems in the elderly. Sleep Medicine Clinics 2006;1: 273–92.
[3] Bachman DL. Sleep disorders with aging: evaluation and treatment. Geriatrics 1992;47(9): 53–6, 59–61.
[4] Bliwise DL. Sleep disorders in Alzheimer's disease and other dementias. Clin Cornerstone 2004;5,6(Suppl 1A):S16–28.
[5] Gaugler JE, Edwards AB, Femia EE, et al. Predictors of institutionalization of cognitively impaired elders: family help and the timing of placement. J Gerontol B Psychol Sci Soc Sci 2000;55(4):P247–55.

 [6] Pollack CP, Perlick D. Sleep problems and institutionalization of the elderly. J Geriatr Psychiatry Neurol 1991;4:204–10.
 [7] Phillips VL, Diwan S. The incremental effect of dementia-related problem behaviors on the time to nursing home placement in poor, frail, demented older people. J Am Geriatr Soc 2003;51(2):188–93.
 [8] Prinz PN, Vitaliano PP, Vitiello MV, et al. Sleep, EEG and mental function changes in senile dementia of the Alzheimer's type. Neurobiol Aging 1982;3(4):361–70.
 [9] Manabe K, Matsui T, Yamaya M, et al. Sleep patterns and mortality among elderly patients in a geriatric hospital. Gerontology 2000;46:318–22.
[10] Brassington GS, King AC, Bliwise DL. Sleep problems as a risk factor for falls in a sample of community-dwelling adults ages 64–99 years. J Am Geriatr Soc 2000;48:1234–40.
[11] Cricco M, Simonsick EM, Foley DJ. The impact of insomnia on cognitive functioning in older adults. J Am Geriatr Soc 2001;49:1185–9.
[12] McCurry SM, Gibbons LE, Logsdon RG, et al. Anxiety and nighttime behavioral disturbances. Awakenings in patients with Alzheimer's disease. J Gerontol Nurs 2004;30(1):12–20.
[13] Kiely DK, Bergmann MA, Jones RN, et al. Characteristics associated with delirium persistence among newly admitted post-acute facility patients. J Gerontol A Biol Sci Med Sci 2004; 59:344–9.
[14] Schnelle JF, Ouslander JG, Simmons SF, et al. Nighttime sleep and bed mobility among incontinent nursing home residents. J Am Geriatr Soc 1993;41:903–9.
[15] Bazil CW. Effects of antiepileptic drugs on sleep structure: are all drugs equal? CNS Drugs 2003;17(10):719–28.
[16] Kaynak D, Kiziltan G, Kaynak H, et al. Sleep and sleepiness in patients with Parkinson's disease before and after dopaminergic treatment. Eur J Neurol 2005;12:199–207.
[17] Landholt HP, Roth C, Dijk DJ, et al. Late-afternoon ethanol intake affects nocturnal sleep and the sleep EEG in middle-aged men. J Clin Psychopharmacol 1996;16(6):428–36.
[18] Page F, Coleman G, Conduit R. The effect of transdermal nicotine patches on sleep and dreams. Physiol Behav 2006;88(4–5):425–32.
[19] Stoschitzky K, Sakotnik A, Lercher P, et al. Influence of beta-blockers on melatonin release. Eur J Clin Pharmacol 1999;55(2):111–5.
[20] Wooten V. Sleep disorders in geriatric patients. Clin Geriatr Med 1992;8(2):427–39.
[21] Zhang L, Samet J, Caffo B, et al. Cigarette smoking and nocturnal sleep architecture. Am J Epidemiol 2006;164:529–37.
[22] Craig D, Hart DJ, Passmore AP. Genetically increased risk of sleep disruption in Alzheimer's disease. Sleep 2006;29(8):1003–7.
[23] Cummings JL, Mega M, Gray K, et al. The neuropsychiatric inventory: comprehensive assessment of psychopathology in dementia. Neurology 1994;44:2308–14.
[24] Johns MW. Sleepiness, snoring and obstructive sleep apnoea: the Epworth sleepiness scale. Chest 1993;103(1):30–6.
[25] Buysse DJ, Reynolds CF, Monk TH, et al. The Pittsburgh sleep quality index: a new instrument for psychiatric practice and research. Psychiatr Res 1989;28:193–213.
[26] Coleman RM, Miles LE, Guilleminault CC. Sleep-wake disorders in the elderly: polysomnographic analysis. J Am Geriatr Soc 1981;29(7):289–96.
[27] Kamel NS, Gammack JK. Insomnia in the elderly: cause, approach and treatment. Am J Med 2006;119(6):463–9.
[28] Little JT, Satlin A, Sunderland T, et al. Sundown syndrome in severely demented patients with probable Alzheimer's disease. J Geriatr Psychiatry Neurol 1995;8:103–6.
[29] Gallagher-Thomson D, Brooks JO III, Bliwise D. The relations among caregiver stress, "sundowning" symptoms, and cognitive decline in Alzheimer's disease. J Am Geriatr Soc 1992;40(8):807–10.
[30] Fiorentino L, Ancoli-Israel S. Sleep disturbances in nursing home patients. Sleep Med Clin 2006;1:293–8.

[31] Gehrman PR, Martin JL, Schochat T. Sleep-disordered breathing and agitation in institutionalized adults with Alzheimer Disease. Am J Geriatr Psychiatry 2003;11:426–33.

[32] Ancoli-Israel S, Martin JL, Kripke DF, et al. Effect of light treatment on sleep and circadian rhythms in demented nursing home patients. J Am Geriatr Soc 2002;50:282–9.

[33] Ancoli-Israel S, Martin JL, Kripke DF, et al. Effect of light on agitation in institutionalized patients with severe Alzheimer's disease. Am J Geriatr Psychiatry 2003;11:194–203.

[34] McCurry SM, Gibbons LE, Logsdon RG, et al. Nighttime insomnia treatment and education for Alzheimer's disease: a randomized, controlled trial. J Am Geriatr Soc 2005;53(5): 793–802.

[35] McCurry SM, Logsdon RG, Vitiello MV, et al. Treatment of sleep and nighttime disturbances in Alzheimer's disease: a behavior management approach. Sleep Med 2004;5(4): 373–7.

[36] McCurry SM, Ancoli-Israel S. Sleep dysfunction in Alzheimer's disease and other dementias. Curr Treat Options Neurol 2003;5(3):261–72.

[37] Doody RS, Stevens JC, Beck C, et al. Practice parameter: management of dementia (an evidence-based review) Report of the Quality Standards Subcommittee of the American Academy of Neurology. Neurology 2001;56(9):1154–66.

[38] National Center on Sleep Disorders research. 2003 National Sleep Disorders Research Plan. Washington, DC: U.S. Department of Health and Human Services; 2003.

[39] Neubauer DN. Sleep problems in the elderly. Am Fam Physician 1999;59(9):2551–60.

[40] Saha S, Robinson S, Bianco T, et al. Efficacy and comparative effectiveness of off-label use of atypical antipsychotics. Portland (OR): The Southern California/RAND Evidence-based Practice Center, The Agency for Healthcare Research and Quality (AHRQ). The John M. Eisenberg Center; 2007.

[41] Singer C, Trachtenberg RE, Kaye J, et al. A multicenter, placebo-controlled trial of melatonin for sleep disturbance in Alzheimer's disease. Sleep 2003;26(7):893–901.

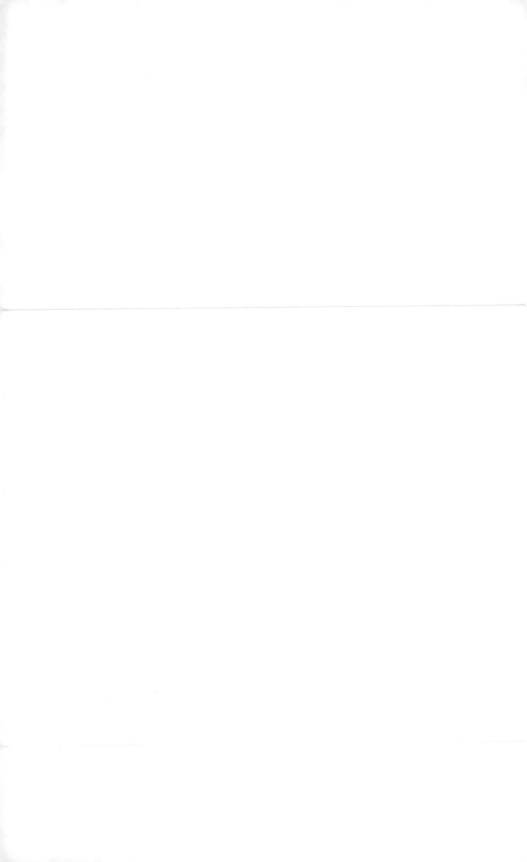

ELSEVIER
SAUNDERS

CLINICS IN
GERIATRIC
MEDICINE

Clin Geriatr Med 24 (2008) 83–91

Sleep Disturbance in Palliative Care

Ramzi R. Hajjar, MD[a,b,*]

[a]*Department of Internal Medicine, Division of Geriatric Medicine,
St. Louis University School of Medicine, 1402 South Grand Boulevard,
Room M238, St. Louis, MO 63104-1028, USA*
[b]*Geriatric Research, Education, and Clinical Center (GRECC),
St. Louis Veterans' Affairs Medical Center,
1 Jefferson Barracks Drive, St. Louis, MO 63125, USA*

Sleep disorders in palliative medicine impose an exceptional challenge to clinicians and an undue burden on patients and their families. Sleep disturbance in patients with terminal conditions differ in several key features from the sleep disorders encountered in the general geriatric population. While primary sleep disorders may occur in patients with terminal conditions, sleep disturbances more commonly develop as a consequence or complication of the terminal condition afflicting the patient, and may consequently have multiple causes. Such sleep disturbances are very common toward the end-of-life, and inflict additional stress on patients already coping with the burden of terminal disease.

At the onset of any discussion on the management of terminal patients, it is prudent to point out the diverse spectrum of patients under palliative care. Diseases qualifying patients for hospice care can broadly be classified as malignant versus nonmalignant (medical) conditions. When the modern hospice movement began in the late 1960s, the caseload predominantly consisted of terminal malignant disease. Today, with the aging of the population, approximately 40% of hospice patients suffer from nonmalignant conditions. Hospice patients will therefore differ vastly in functional capacity, physiologic reserve, physical needs, and expectations. Furthermore, the natural progression of chronic medical conditions follows a course much less consistent or predictable than that for malignant conditions. Consequently, the prevalence of sleep disorders in palliative medicine varies widely based on the definition used, the stage of the disease (eg, Karnofsky score),

* Department of Internal Medicine, Division of Geriatric Medicine, St. Louis University Health Sciences Center, 1402 South Grand Boulevard, Room M238, St. Louis, MO 63104-1028.
  E-mail address: hajjarrr@aol.com

0749-0690/08/$ - see front matter. Published by Elsevier Inc.
doi:10.1016/j.cger.2007.08.003

and the disease process, and has been estimated at 22% to 100% [1,2]. The impact on quality of life could potentially be immense because some patients may survive many months or years with chronic, albeit progressive, diseases. Conditions in which somatic or psychosocial stressors result in disruption of sleep will clearly affect the quality of life during wakeful hours.

The goal in managing any symptomatic condition in the hospice and palliative model of care shifts from a curative and preventive approach to one of palliation and symptom management. The management of sleep disorders is no exception. Such a paradigm shift is often difficult to embrace unless the health care provider is accomplished in delivering care to dying patients, and the patients and their social support are accepting of the inevitable progression of the disease process and the futility of aggressive tertiary intervention (Table 1). Curative and palliative models of care, however, need not be mutually exclusive; in fact, they work best in conjunction with each other.

Comprehensive management of sleep disturbances involves addressing medical and psychosocial causes contributing to the problem, as well as treating the symptom as an entity in itself. In other words, the treatment goal becomes symptom management, independent of the effect on disease progression or outcome. As such, quality of life becomes the substitute measure of treatment success. The stated goal of the National Hospice Organization best depicts the duality approach to care:

Table 1
Curative and palliative models of care

	Curative care	Palliative care
1. Goal	Primary goal is cure	Primary goal is relief of suffering
2. Investigation	Object of analysis is the disease process	Object of analysis is the patient and family
3. Object of investigation	Primary value is placed on measurable data	Measurable and subjective data are valued
4. Symptom management	Symptoms are treated primarily as clues to diagnosis	Distressing symptoms are treated as entities in themselves
5. Subjective assessment	Devaluates subjective or unverifiable information	Values the patient's experience of an illness
6. Indication for therapy	Therapy is indicated if it slows or eradicates the disease process	Therapy is indicated if it controls symptoms and relieves suffering
7. Holistic approach	The patient's body is differentiated from the mind	Patients are seen as complex beings with physical, emotional, social, and spiritual dimensions
8. End-point	Death is the ultimate failure	Enabling a patient to live fully and comfortably until he or she dies is a success

The hospice philosophy of care affirms support and care for people in the last phases of incurable disease so that they may live as full and as comfortably as possible. Hospice recognizes dying as part of the normal process of living and focuses on maintaining the quality of remaining life. Hospice affirms life and neither hastens nor postpones death. Hospice exists in the hope and belief that through appropriate care, and the promotion of a caring community sensitive to their needs, patients and their families may be free to attain a degree of mental and spiritual preparation for death that is satisfactory to them [3].

The potential long-term complications of treating sleep disorders in this population must be weighed against the subjective and immediate benefit, as determined by the patient, and will often play a lesser role in guiding optimal therapy. For example, the increased risk of traumatic falls with the use of sedating hypnotics is a debatable concern in a frail terminal patient who will imminently be bedridden. Proper care clearly will differ greatly among patients, and is made more arduous by the subjective rather than objective measure of success. Therein lies the challenge of quality palliative care: to manage symptoms without advancing the disease process. Because addressing either of these is likely to affect the other, a delicate balance must be struck between antipathetic forces, which overlap at times and conflict at others. With sleep disorders in terminal patients, such a balance is not always easy to achieve, because symptom management and perception of disease progression are typically in sharp contrast. A common unifying concept that can be offered to patients and their families, once the finality of the inevitable outcome is accepted, is hope—not for a cure, but for the absence of suffering at the end of life.

Despite the tremendous benefit in managing this potentially treatable condition, few health care providers aggressively pursue sleep symptoms in terminally ill patients. Similarly, few patients report these symptoms as being problematic. For some, it is viewed as an inevitable consequence of the terminal condition. Others may view the sleep disorders as a lesser disturbance when compared with the burden of the disease, or may not identify it as an independent problem. While much has been published on sleep disorders associated with specific chronic disease entities, surprisingly little data exist as to the overall management of sleep disorders in terminal patients under the rubric of broader hospice principles [4]. This article reviews some unique features of sleep disorders as they relate to general principles of hospice care. For a more detailed disease-specific review, by Martin and Ancoli-Israel elsewhere in this issue, or in other excellent reviews [2].

Common contributing causes of sleep disorders and their assessment

Pain is a leading quality-of-life determinant at the end of life that is often inadequately treated. It is estimated that up to 90% of cancer patients experience significant pain during the course of their disease [5,6]. Furthermore, approximately one third of cancer patients reported pain that interfered with sleep onset, while two thirds complained of difficulty maintaining sleep through the night because of pain [7,8]. One study showed pain intensity to correlate inversely with total hours of sleep in cancer patients [9]. While pain is commonly thought of as a feature of malignant disease, nonmalignant conditions are often associated with significant pain as well. In fact, non-cancer patients did not differ from cancer patients in the incidence and severity of pain in one small study [10]. Other factors that must be considered in the management of pain include how sleep deprivation effects pain threshold and perception, and how psychologic factors, such as anxiety and depression, modify the sleep-pain relationship. Numerous pharmacologic, as well as and nonpharmacologic, options are available for pain management. Any of these modalities can be employed independently or in combination to achieve optimal pain control. Optimal control is often subjectively determined by the patient, and is decided by many factors, including pain threshold, effect of pain on sleep, and acceptable levels of iatrogenic sedation. It has been shown that adequate pain management improves the duration and quality of sleep [11,12]. In a validation study of pain management, the mean total sleep time as much as doubled in cancer patients treated for pain, according to the World Health Organization guidelines [13].

Depression is another condition commonly encountered in palliative medicine that is under-diagnosed and, when diagnosed, under-treated. Depression may be worsened by sleep deprivation and pain, and in turn may itself worsen these two conditions. The prevalence of depression varies widely, based on the criteria used to establish the diagnosis as well as the stage of the disease. The prevalence has ranged from 8% to 58% in various terminal patient cohorts [2]. Sleep disturbance is a hallmark of depression, and the prevalence statistics indicate that depression seriously impacts sleep in the terminally ill. For this reason, it is surprising that antidepressants are administered so infrequently. In a study by Bukberg and colleagues [14], 42% of hospitalized cancer patients met criteria for depression but only 6% were receiving antidepressants. There has been ample room to debate the distinction between "normal" grief and clinical depression, and the efficacy of antidepressants in the acute management of depression-induced insomnia. Reactive or situational depression, as a response to a terminal diagnosis, is viewed by many as being a normal stage of grieving, and therefore does not warrant treatment, which, in part, explains the low treatment frequency. Grief is more often addressed with anxiolytics, which are not intended for chronic use because of the development of rapid tolerance, and which do little toward alleviating the more persistent depression many terminal patients will experience.

Cognitive impairment, particularly delirium, and to a lesser extent dementia, disrupt the sleep-wake cycle and are common among terminally ill patients [15,16]. In its early stages, delirium may go unrecognized or be mistaken for anxiety or depression, or attributed to organ failure or other physiologic decline. Treatment includes eliminating the cause when possible, and the use of appropriate hypnotic medications in delirium. Pharmacologic management of cognitive impairment must be exercised with the knowledge that the medications themselves are not an uncommon cause of delirium.

Many other physical ailments contribute to sleep disorders in terminally ill patients. These include respiratory distress, gastrointestinal disorders, and nutritional disorders. Iatrogenic etiologies include medication, disruption of sleep routine, and hospitalization. Medications that effect sleep include those that interfere with sleep as well as those that cause over-sedation and excessive sleep. Several studies have documented the sleep disruption that occurs with hospital admission [17,18]. The environment and daily routine of terminal patients should be kept as constant as possible. Many terminal patients report better quality of sleep at home, despite less aggressive disease management, when compared with institutionalized patients.

Nonpharmacologic management of sleep disorders

Sleep can be improved by a variety of pharmacologic and nonpharmacologic intervention. Nonpharmacologic interventions often tend to be overlooked or abandoned because of the ease of drug intervention and the abundance of medications available for this goal. Significant sleep improvement can be achieved with cognitive-behavioral intervention and sleep hygiene. Appropriate sleep depends on psychophysiologic (internal) and environmental (external) circumstances, both of which can be modified with skillful intervention. The effectiveness of cognitive and behavioral interventions vary but are promising, and no single approach has been shown to be the most effective. Successful application of behavioral modification depends on appropriately matching the treatment modality with the patient needs.

Basic sleep hygiene principles, as discussed in other articles, can be applied to most palliative patients, particularly early in the course of their disease. These common-sense guidelines are effective and easy to comprehend, yet few patients adhere to them and many clinicians detract or discount them in favor of pharmacologic intervention. In terminal patients, daytime activity is often substantially curtailed, and a blurring of the wake-sleep cycle develops, particularly when the daytime routine involves prolonged periods of recumbency. Nighttime mind-racing, anxiety, agitation, and restlessness result in extended nonrestful periods of time in bed, which in itself becomes a source of frustration. Awareness of the elapsing time and watching the clock only adds to the pressure to fall asleep. In such situations, patients should get out of bed when able, and participate in a relaxing activity, such as reading or watching television, until the feeling of somnolence returns. Daytime physical activity, in as much as permitted by the disease process, is helpful in promoting sleep at night; however, exercise should be avoided in the immediate hours before sleep because of the stimulation which may interfere with the onset of sleep. Similarly, sleep restriction during the day will prolong the period of time patients sleep during the night. L-Tryptophan, an essential amino acid found in dairy products and other food stuff, has been investigated as a naturally occurring sedating sleep aid, but its clinical effect is inconsistent and modest [19]. Stimulants such as caffeine, tobacco, and in some cases alcohol should be avoided before sleep.

Cognitive-behavioral intervention has emerged as a mainstay in the management of chronic insomnia associated with heightened cognitive or physiologic arousal [2]. Numerous techniques have been employed in the cognitive-behavioral approach to insomnia. A successful intervention depends on appropriate patient selection, and matching patients to the proper intervention or combination of interventions. Although time consuming and demanding, and requiring some effort on behalf of the patient and provider, good results have been reported with techniques such as biofeedback and progressive muscle relaxation. In one small study, a significant reduction in sleep latency and increase in total sleep time was reported after only three days of relaxation training [20]. Other meta-analysis does not indicate progressive muscle relaxation to be highly effective when used as a sole intervention [21,22], but may be an important component of feedback intervention. Biofeedback is a useful technique in teaching patients how to achieve a state of relaxation inductive to sleep. It must be matched with specific patient need, and may include input from diverse systems, such as mental imaging, skin conduction, muscle tension, and vasomotor tone, all with the ultimate goal of alleviating psychophysiologic arousal.

Perhaps the intervention most consistently found to be effective, when feasible, is sleep restriction. Many terminal patients spend significant amount of wakeful (though not necessarily restful) time in bed during the day. An unhealthy association between recumbency and insomnia develops, and over time the mere thought of the bed and sleep arouses feelings of tension and arousal. Limiting the amount of time a person spends in bed while awake will greatly increase the onset, duration, and quality of sleep during nighttime [23]. In early stages, sleep deprivation can be stressful to some patients and may initially cause increased sleep disturbances. Daytime sleep restriction may not be appropriate for some terminally ill patients, with disease burden often being the determining factor.

Pharmacologic management of sleep disorders

Because many terminal patients with insomnia are unable to participate actively in nonpharmacologic modalities, and in many cases these modalities are insufficient to achieve the desired restful state, hypnotic medications are frequently used to achieve this goal. Concerns with these medications in the general geriatric population, such as tolerance, dose escalation, over sedation, physical and psychologic dependency, and risk of falls and cognitive impairment (among other adverse reactions), become less relevant in palliative care patients where life expectancy is limited and the primary goal of treatment is symptomatic relief. Once initiated, long-term use is usually necessary, though short-term or intermittent use remains the preferred method of use to minimize accumulation of serum drug levels and physiologic tolerance.

Many classes of medications have been used in the management of insomnia in terminal patients (see the article by Tariq and Pulisetty, elsewhere in this issue). The general principles of pharmacologic management of insomnia in palliative care mirror those of the general geriatric population, with the added challenge of diverse and rapidly diminishing physiologic reserve. The choice of medication must be predicated by achieving a delicate balance between desired clinical response and adverse effect. Metabolism of most hypnotic medications is diminished in the frail and infirm elderly. Even at comparable serum levels, the elderly have increased sensitivity to hypnotics when compared with the young [2]. Dosing regimens must reflect this sensitivity to both desired effect as well as side effects. With most medications, it may be prudent to initiate therapy at half the smallest recommended dose, and advance the treatment as needed. Short-acting drugs administered before bedtime result in less daytime sedation and are the accepted standard of care, but are also more commonly associated with rebound insomnia following abrupt withdrawal of medication. On the other hand, long-acting hypnotics may have a daytime carry-over anxiolytic effect that may be beneficial in some terminally ill patients. Anticholinergic side effects, particularly with the sedating antidepressants, must also be considered during drug selection, and symptoms such as delirium and urinary retention must be monitored and addressed. Furthermore, because insomnia in palliative care is often the result of clinical manifestation of advanced-stage disease, aggressive pharmacologic management of all symptoms contributing to sleep disturbance must be addressed. These include psychologic symptoms, such as depression and anxiety, as well as physical symptoms, such as dyspnea, gastroesophageal reflux, and pain.

Benzodiazepines remain the standard initial medications of choice for the management of short-term insomnia in terminal patients. They are effective in reducing sleep latency and prolonging total sleep, and are relatively well tolerated when used appropriately. The efficacy and safety of long term benzodiazepine use remains debatable. Newer preparations are presumably well tolerated chronically and are less likely to induce tolerance. Sedating tricyclic antidepressants (TCA) have been used successfully in the management of insomnia. When effective, they can be used chronically without the concern of physiologic tolerance or addiction. Anticholinergic side effects are common, and the relatively long half-life and potential for overdose and toxicity make patient selection of particular importance when considering these drugs for therapy. Secondary amine TCAs produce less anticholinergic side effects but are also less sedating. The sedating heterocyclic antidepressant, trazodone, has a shorter half life than most TCAs and milder anticholinergic side effects, making it the preferred drug of choice. Starting dose is typically 50 mg daily, and may be titrated up to 300 mg daily if needed. With continued use, sedating antidepressants have the added benefits of treating anxiety and depression, commonly encountered in terminally ill patients, as well as possibly ameliorating the pain threshold. The newer generation antidepressants, such as mirtazapine and nefazodone, though sedating, are primarily used for management of depression. Barbiturates have fallen out of favor because of the rapid development of tolerance and their narrow safety margin. Finally, melatonin has been widely used for sleep promotion, but no large-scale controlled study has demonstrated its effectiveness in the management of insomnia. It has been shown to be of value, however, in the management of phase shifts in the wake-sleep cycle [24,25].

Summary

Sleep disorders are very common in palliative medicine and may tremendously affect the quality of life of patients already burdened by terminal illness. It is important to screen terminal patients for sleep disorders, and realize that insomnia is not an inevitable untreatable consequence of the dying process. It is the duty of the health care provider to proactively inquire about sleep disturbances, because many terminally ill patients will not report them or identify them as an independent problem. Sleep pathology in palliative care often stems from the terminal disease condition, but primary sleep disorders and sleep disturbances caused by anxiety and depression are also common. Whatever the cause, sleep disturbance should be viewed as an entity in itself, and the goal of treatment centered around improving the quality of life despite the progressing underlying illness. In many cases, sleep quality can be improved with pharmacologic and non-pharmacologic interventions, requiring the concerted effort of the provider, patient, and caregiver.

References

[1] Huge L, Ellershaw JE, Cook L, et al. The prevalence, key causes and management of insomnia in palliative care patients. J Pain Symptom Manage 2004;27:316–21.
[2] Sateia MJ, Santulli RB. Sleep in palliative care. In: Doyle D, Hanks G, Cherny NI, et al, editors. Oxford textbook of palliative medicine. New York: Oxford University Press; 2004. p. 731–46.
[3] National Hospice Organization. Standards of a Hospice Program of Care. page iii. Arlington (VA): 1993.

[4] Gibson J, Grealish L. Relating palliative care principles to the promotion of undisturbed sleep in a hospice setting. Int J Palliat Nurs 2001;7:140–5.
[5] Bonica JJ. Importance of the problem. In: Bonica JJ, Ventafridda V, editors. Advances in Pain Research and Therapy. Vol 2. New York: Raven Press; 1979. p. 1–12.
[6] Twycross RG, Fairfields S. Pain in far advanced cancer. Pain 1982;14:303–10.
[7] Banning A, Sjogren P, Henriksen H. Pain causes in 200 patients referred to a multidisciplinary cancer pain clinic. Pain 1991;45:45–8.
[8] Dorrepaal KL, Aaronson NK, Van Dam FS. Pain experience and pain management among hospitalized cancer patients. A clinical study. Cancer 1989;63:593–8.
[9] Tamburini M, Selmi S, de Conno F, et al. Semantic descriptors of pain. Pain 1987;29:187–93.
[10] Donovan MI, Dillon P, McGuire L. Incidence and characteristics of pain in a sample of medical-surgical patients. Pain 1987;30:69–78.
[11] Hanks GW, Twycross RG, Bliss JM. Controlled release morphine tablets: a double-blind trial in patients with advanced cancer. Anaesthesia 1987;42:840–4.
[12] Lapin J, Portenoy RK, Coyle N, et al. Guidelines for use of controlled-release morphine in cancer pain management. Cancer Nurs 1989;12:202–8.
[13] Ventafridda V, Tamburini M, Caraceni A, et al. A validation study of the WHO method for cancer pain relief. Cancer 1987;59:850–6.
[14] Bukberg J, Penman D, Holland JC. Depression in hospitalized cancer patients. Psychosom Med 1984;46:199–212.
[15] Derogatiss LR, Morrow GR, Fetting J, et al. The prevalence of psychiatric disorders among cancer patents. J Am Med Assoc 1983;249:751–7.
[16] Massie MJ, Holland J, Glass E. Delirium in terminally ill cancer patients. Am J Psychiatry 1983;140:1048–50.
[17] Broughton R, Baron R. Sleep of acute coronary patients in an open ward type intensive care unit. Sleep Research 1973;2:144.
[18] Topf M, Thompson S. Interactive relationships hospital patients' noise-induced stress and other stress with sleep. Heart Lung 2001;30:237–43.
[19] Hartmann E. L-Tryptophan: a rational hypnotic with clinical potential. Am J Psychiatry 1977;134:366–70.
[20] Cannici J, Malcom R, Peck LA. Treatment of insomnia in cancer patients using muscle relaxation training. J Behav Ther Exp Psychiatry 1983;14:251–6.
[21] Morin CM, Culbert JP, Schwartz SM. Nonpharmacological interventions for insomnia: a meta-analysis of treatment efficacy. Am J Psychiatry 1994;151:1172–80.
[22] Murtagh DR, Greenwood KM. Identifying effective psychological treatments for insomnia: a meta-analysis. J Consult Clin Psychol 1995;63:79–89.
[23] Spielman AJ, Saskin P, Thorpy MJ. Treatment of chronic insomnia byrestriction of time in bed. Sleep 1987;10:45–56.
[24] Attenburrow ME, Dowling BA, Sargent PA, et al. Melatonin phase advances circadian rhythm. Psychopharmacology (Berl) 1995;121:503–5.
[25] Dawson D, Encel N, Lushington K. Improving adaptation to simulated night shift: time exposure to bright light versus daytime melatonin administration. Sleep 1995;18:11–21.

ELSEVIER
SAUNDERS

CLINICS IN
GERIATRIC
MEDICINE

Clin Geriatr Med 24 (2008) 93–105

Pharmacotherapy for Insomnia

Syed H. Tariq, MD, FACP*, Shailaja Pulisetty, MD

*Department of Internal Medicine, Division of Geriatrics, Saint Louis University School
of Medicine, 1402 So. Grand Boulevard M-238, Saint Louis, MO 63104, USA*

Since the mid 1800s, a variety of medications have become available for the treatment of insomnia. Bromide was the first agent used as sedative hypnotic, followed by chloral hydrate, paraldehyde, and urethane. Chloral hydrate has a half-life of 4 to 8 hours and is an effective hypnotic with a rapid onset of action. The main disadvantages of this medication include a rapid onset of tolerance and a very narrow therapeutic window.

Barbiturates were introduced in the early 1900s, by the 1960s they constituted about 55% of hypnotic prescriptions [1]. Barbiturates increase total sleep time, reduce sleep latency, and reduce the duration of rapid eye movement (REM). Tolerance develops rapidly and upon abrupt discontinuation many users experience rebound effects, including nightmares. In the 1970s, several benzodiazepines became available and quickly became the agents of choice for insomnia treatment. In the last two decades, several new pharmacologic classes for insomnia have been introduced and are quickly replacing benzodiazepines.

Although hypnotics are the most common treatment for insomnia at all ages, usage is disproportionately high in older adults. Community use rates for hypnotics among adults over age 65 range from 3% to 21% for men, and 7% to 29% for women [2], compared with only 2% to 4% for younger age groups [3]. An observational study compared insomnia patients to matched samples without insomnia, 75,558 elderly patients with insomnia, plus equal-sized, matched comparison groups. The direct cost considered included inpatient, outpatient, pharmacy, and emergency room costs for all diseases for 6 months. Indirect costs included costs related to absenteeism from work and the use of short-term disability programs. Among the elderly, direct costs were about $1,143 greater for insomnia patients. This study suggests that insomnia is associated with a significant economic burden for older patients [4].

---

* Corresponding author.
E-mail address: tariqsh@slu.edu (S.H. Tariq).

0749-0690/08/$ - see front matter © 2008 Elsevier Inc. All rights reserved.
doi:10.1016/j.cger.2007.08.009   *geriatric.theclinics.com*

Unfortunately, pharmacologic studies of insomnia in the elderly are scarce and the magnitude of medication benefit is frequently unimpressive. Medication side effects, such as falls, confusion, dizziness, and headache continue to be of concern in this frail population. An ideal hypnotic agent has been characterized to have rapid onset of action and elimination, improved ability to initiate and maintain sleep, improved sleep quality, improved daytime performance, minimal drug interactions, absent hangover effects, and no significant potential for tolerance, abuse, dependence, and withdrawal or rebound effects [5,6]. At this time, a variety of medicines are used for the treatment of insomnia because of their hypnotic or sedative properties. Most have one or more unwanted cognitive side effects, which in the elderly can result in confusion, dizziness, and falls. As the search for an ideal hypnotic continues, it will be important to learn more about the function of sleep at a cellular and molecular level.

The Food and Drug Administration (FDA) has approved numerous agents for insomnia treatment. These medications include benzodiazepines (flurazepam, triazolam, quazepam, estazolam, temazepam) and nonbenzodiazepines (zolpidem, zaleplon, eszopiclone, ramelteon). These agents are all indicated for short-term usage with the exception of eszopiclone. The properties and side effects of these drugs, those that are commonly used but not FDA approved for insomnia, and are available over-the-counter, are outlined in Table 1.

Pharmacotherapy of insomnia in the elderly may be complicated by age related changes in pharmacodynamics and pharmacokinetics. The general rule of initiating medications should also be applied for agent use in the treatment of insomnia: start low and go slow. Insomnia therapy ideally consists of behavioral therapy and pharmacotherapy with approved agents. This article only discusses the pharmacologic approach to the treatment of insomnia in older adults.

Pharmacologic categories

Benzodiazepine receptor agonists

All benzodiazepine (BZD) receptor agonists have been shown to improve sleep quality by reducing the latency of sleep onset, nocturnal awakening, and REM sleep. With varying half-lives and duration of action, these agents reduce the likelihood of arousing during sleep, thereby allowing increased total sleep time. With aging there is increase in body fat mass, and thus increased amount of unbound drug and increase half-life. Thus benzodiazepines with a long half-life should be avoided [7]. Rebound insomnia can occur with cessation of use after only 1 to 2 weeks of treatment. There is also a risk of developing tolerance, addiction, and daytime sleepiness to benzodiazepines [8]. Accidents are reported with agents with a long half-life or in patients with prolonged impaired sleep secondary to long-term use [9].

The BZD mechanism of action is via gamma-aminobutyric acid (GABA) receptor complex inhibition through occupation of the available binding subunits (ie, the BZD receptor). GABA receptors are present throughout the brain, including the ventral lateral preoptic area that controls sleep. Temazepam is the most commonly used BZD hypnotic, with a half-life of 8 to 25 hours, and can be given in dosages from 7.5 mg to 30 mg at night [10]. In a small study of older adults, temazapam 7.5 mg was evaluated in a sleep laboratory using a 2-week protocol. It was concluded from the study that in older adults short term use of temazapam was effective and there were minimum adverse effects [11]. A meta-analysis of sedative-hypnotics versus benzodiazepines was conducted and included 24 studies and 2,417 subjects [12]. Mild sleep benefits were seen, with both groups showing increased sleep time of 25 to 34 minutes and decreased number of awakenings per night; however, side effects, especially central nervous system symptoms, was increased in both treatment groups. The number needed to treat for any sleep benefit was 13 and the number needed to harm for any side effect was 6. In general, there was no difference in side effects between the sedative-hypnotics and the benzodiazepines.

A prospective 5-year study looked at the risk of injury associated with the use of various benzodiazepines. The study included a total of 253,244 community-dwellers aged 65 years and older, who were nonusers of benzodiazepines at the beginning of the observation period. Benzodiazepines with intermediate, long, and very long half-life were used in this study. Twenty eight percent received one or more prescriptions of benzodiazepine and 18% sustained one of more injury, of which 50% were fractures. Higher-dose equivalents of oxazepam, flurazepam, and chlordiazepoxide were associated with the greatest risk for injury. The risks for injury with the current use of benzodiazepines, compared with nonuse periods in the same subject, varied according to the type of benzodiazepine but did not correlate with half-life and were associated with an increased risk for injuries [13].

Another meta-analysis (mean duration of treatment 2.2 weeks, 24 randomized control trials, age range 58 to 98 years) showed that participants who received sedatives had slightly better sleep quality, longer total sleep time, and fewer night awakenings than did those who received placebo; results were similar when benzodiazepines were compared with placebo. Participants who received sedatives had higher risk for cognitive adverse events and reported more morning or daytime fatigue than did those who received placebo (seven randomized controlled trials, n = 829), but groups did not differ for psychomotor adverse events. Four trials (n = 1,072) showed that 13 patients would need to be treated with a sedative for one additional patient to have an improvement in sleep quality. Sixteen trials (n = 2,220) showed that six patients would need to be treated for one additional patient to have an adverse effect [14].

Table 1
Commonly used medications for insomnia

Class	Agent	Dose (mg)	Half life (h)	Receptor	Year approved	Side effects	Comments
Benzodiazepine	Flurazepam	15–30	50–100	GABA-BZD	1970	Dizziness, drowsiness, ataxia, amnesia, falls, gastrointestinal upset	FDA approved for insomnia; abuse potential; rebound insomnia; tolerance and dependence; hangover effect; increased fall risk; cytochrome P450 metabolism
	Estazolam	0.5–2	10–24	GABA-BZD	1980		
	Temazepam	7.5–30	8–25	GABA-BZD	1981		
	Triazolam	0.125–0.25	1.5–5.5	GABA-BZD	1982		
	Quazepam	7.5–15	39–73	GABA-BZD	1985		
Sedative-Hypnotics	Zolpidem	5–20	2.5–2.8	GABA-A: alpha-1	1993	Dizziness, drowsiness, amnesia, headache, gastrointestinal upset	For sleep-onset insomnia; risk of dependence & rebound; abuse potential
	Zaleplon	5–10	1.0	GABA-A: omega 1	1997	Headache, dizziness, myalgia, amnesia	For sleep-onset insomnia; no tolerance or hangover
	Eszopiclone	1–3	5–7	GABA-A	2004	Dry mouth, unpleasant taste, dizziness, amnesia, gastrointestinal upset	Studied in elderly; favorable side-effect profile; FDA approved for long-term use

Class	Drug	Dose	Half-life	Mechanism	Year	Side effects	Comments
Melatonin receptor agonist	Ramelteon	8	1.5	MT1, MT2	2005	Fatigue, dizziness, headache, nausea	Studied in elderly; favorable side-effect profile
Antidepressants	Trazodone	50–150	Early: 3–6 Late: 5–9	Possible: 5-HT2	1981	Antidepressant, dry mouth, dizziness, headache, nervousness, orthostasis	Not FDA approved for insomnia; primary use: depression
	Amitriptyline Doxepin	10–100 75–150	12–24 Early: 17 Late: 52	5-HT2 noradrenaline Postsynaptic: H1, H2, Alpha-1, 5-HT2, muscarinic	1961 1969	Dry mouth, dizziness, QTc prolongation, constipation, orthostasis	Not FDA approved for insomnia; narrow therapeutic window; anticholinergic side-effects; cardiotoxic; overdose potential
	Trimipramine	25–100	11–23	Postsynaptic: H1, H2, Alpha-1, 5-HT2, muscarinic	1982		
Nonprescription	Diphenhydramine	25–50	2–9	Antihistamine: H-1	1946	Drowsiness, dry mouth, dizziness, constipation	Not FDA approved for insomnia; anticholinergic side-effects
	Melatonin	1–3	1–2	Melatonin		Headache, irritability, dizziness	No quality controls; not FDA-regulated
	Valerian	400–900	1–2	Possible: GABA-A, adenosine, 5HT-5a		Headache, restlessness, gastrointestinal upset	No quality controls; not FDA-regulated

Abbreviations: BZD, benzodiazepine; GABA, gamma-aminobutyric acid; H1, histamine; MT, melatonin; 5HT-2 serotonin type 2 receptor antagonism.

Nonbenzodiazepines

Unlike benzodiazepines, nonbenzodiazepines show relative specificity for one or more of the GABA subtypes. Because of lower incidence of retrograde amnesia, daytime sleepiness, respiratory depression, and orthostatic hypotension, the nonBZDs have become more popular than BZD for insomnia therapy.

Zolpidem

Zolpidem selectively binds to the alpha-1 subunit of GABA receptors. Zolpidem has a rapid onset of action and a short half-life (2.5–2.8 hours), making it more useful in sleep onset insomnia rather than for improving sleep maintenance [10]. Zolpidem produces strong sedative effect without the anxiolytic, muscle relaxant, and anticonvulsant effects seen with BZDs [15]. Unlike the benzodiazepines, zolpidem does not alter the normal sleep architecture and there is no reported REM sleep suppression. Zolpidem is metabolized primarily by the cytochrome isoenzyme 3A4, unlike the benzodiazepines that are metabolized by several cytochrome P450 isoenzymes, resulting in fewer drug-drug interactions. Zolpidem is available in both short- and long-acting preparations.

Zolpidem is being assessed for its efficacy and tolerability in 119 elderly psychiatric in-patients with insomnia. Zolpidem (20 mg/d) significantly improved total duration of sleep at 28 days compared with placebo. When 10 mg/d or 20 mg/d zolpidem were compared, there was also a trend toward improvement in all other sleep parameters. Daytime drowsiness was reported in three patients receiving 20 mg/d zolpidem compared with one receiving 10 mg/d zolpidem. This study concluded that in elderly psychiatric patients, 10 mg/d zolpidem can be used to treat insomnia and can be safely added to concomitant psychotropic treatment without inducing daytime drowsiness [16]. The most common side effects include nausea, dizziness, and drowsiness [17]. It is contraindicated in sleep-related breathing disorders [10], severe hepatic impairment, acute pulmonary impairment, and respiratory depression [17]. Unlike zaleplon, zolpidem is associated with dependence and has the potential for abuse [18].

Zaleplon

Zaleplon is a short-acting (elimination half-life of 1 hour), nonBZD hypnotic that acts on the benzodiazepine type 1 site of the GABA-A receptor complex. Zaleplon increases total sleep time and decreases awakenings. Zaleplon has a short half-life of one hour and is not associated with tolerance or rebound insomnia or hangover. Zaleplon reduced sleep latency and sleep quality, but these results were based only on self-reports. It is effective in both 5-mg and 10-mg doses [19]. Zaleplon is reported to be safe and efficacious in both short- and long-term use in older adults [20,21].

Eszopiclone

Eszopiclone is the first hypnotic agent for which a long-term, randomized, double blind, placebo controlled study has been performed. It is approved for treatment of sleep onset and sleep maintenance insomnia. Escopiclone, works by binding the GABA-A receptor. In a randomized controlled trial of 264 older adults, escopiclone showed a significant reduction in sleep latency of 27 minutes and increased total sleep time of 49 minutes when compared with placebo [22].

In another randomized trial (n = 231) of older adults, the eszopiclone 2-mg group had a significantly shorter sleep latency compared with placebo. The eszopiclone 2-mg group had significantly longer total sleep time and eszopiclone 1-mg group had significantly shorter sleep latency compared with placebo. It was concluded from this study that nightly treatment with eszopiclone 1 mg effectively induced sleep, while the 2-mg dose was effective in inducing and maintaining sleep. Eszopiclone was well tolerated in elderly patients with primary insomnia [23]. Eszopiclone has longer half-life than other nonBZD. It has been shown to decrease sleep latency and wake time after sleep onset and increased sleep efficiency for 6 months compared with placebo in two multicenter trials [24,25].

In the trials of elderly patients, who received eszopiclone 2 mg or placebo for 2 weeks, eszopiclone was associated with significantly shorter sleep latency compared with placebo, as well as a significant decrease in the cumulative number of naps. The most commonly reported drug-related, dose-responsive adverse event in clinical trials of eszopiclone 2 and 3 mg was bitter taste (17% and 34%, respectively), followed by dizziness (5% and 7%) and dry mouth (5% and 7%). Somnolence occurred at an incidence of 4% to 9% with both doses. Tolerance or rebound insomnia was not reported [26]. The recent National Institutes of Health (NIH) State-of-the-Science conference on insomnia concluded that benzodiazepine-receptor actives (BzRAs) are efficacious in the short-term management of insomnia, and the frequency and severity of adverse effects are much lower in the newer nonbenzodiazepine BzRAs [27]. All other medications that are prescribed for insomnia (eg, sedating antidepressants, antihistamines) are used off label.

Ramelteon

The most recently released insomnia medication, ramelteon, acts as a melatonin receptor agonist. Ramelteon is high selective to melatonin (MT) 1 and MT2 receptors in the suprachiasmatic nucleus of the hypothalamus. It improves latency to persistent sleep and total sleep time in adults with transient and chronic insomnia, and in elderly with chronic insomnia [28]. Ramelteon is contraindicated in patients taking fluvoxamine and should be used with caution in patients with coexisting depression. Because liver metabolizes ramelteon, it should not be prescribed to patients with hepatic insufficiency. The advantages of ramelteon, when compared with other available hypnotics, are that it is nonscheduled medication and it can be safely used for long-term treatment of insomnia without any potential for abuse or dependence. In a month-long study of older adults (mean age 72 years) with chronic primary insomnia, ramelteon reduced sleep latency by 8 minutes and total sleep time was increased by 12 minutes [29]. Although no rebound or withdrawal symptoms are reported with ramelteon, the clinical relevance of these benefits should been considered.

When all the nonBZDs are compared with placebo it appears that they are effective at improving sleep latency and sleep quality, and least effective at enhancing total sleep time. The efficacy of ramelteon is limited to improving sleep latency, while all other agents, especially at higher doses, were found to produce improvement in both sleep latency and some improvement in total sleep time. Based on the limited data available in older adults, zopiclone, zolpidem, zaleplon, eszopiclone, and ramelteon represent modestly effective and generally well-tolerated treatments for insomnia [30].

In a review of the literature from 1996 to 2006, all options available for the treatment of chronic insomnia were considered. Most of these studies were of short duration and did not enroll exclusively older adults. Compared with the benzodiazepines, the non-benzodiazepine sedative-hypnotics appeared to offer few, if any, significant clinical advantages in efficacy or tolerability in older adults. It was concluded that long-term use of sedative-hypnotics for insomnia lacks an evidence base and has been discouraged for reasons such as potential adverse drug effects as cognitive impairment (anterograde amnesia), daytime sedation, motor incoordination, and increased risk of motor vehicle accidents and falls. In addition, the effectiveness and safety of long-term use of these agents remain to be determined [31].

Antidepressants

All of the antidepressants except trazodone suppress REM sleep. Unlike GABA agonists, antidepressants have less pronounced effect on sleep induction. Mechanisms explaining the sedative effect of antidepressants include histamine (H 1), serotonin type 2 (5HT2) receptor antagonism, and possibly alpha1-adrenergic receptor antagonism.

Trazadone, a triazolopyridine antidepressant, is currently the second most commonly prescribed agent for the treatment of insomnia because of its sedating qualities. A review of 18 trials suggests that evidence for the efficacy of trazadone in treating insomnia is very limited; most studies are small and conducted in populations of depressed patients. Side effects associated with trazadone are sedation, dizziness, and psychomotor impairment, which raise particular concern regarding its use in the elderly. There is also some evidence of tolerance related to use of trazadone [32].

There is little data to suggest that trazodone improves sleep in patients without mood disorder, though it does increase total sleep in patients with major depressive disorder [33]. In clinical practice, low doses of sedating antidepressant medications often are used to treat insomnia, even in the nondepressed individual. The NIH State-of-the-Science conference on insomnia concluded that in short-term use, trazodone is sedating and improves several sleep parameters, but these initial effects may not last beyond 2 weeks. There are, however, no long-term studies of trazodone for the treatment of insomnia. Doxepin has been found to have beneficial effects on sleep for up to 4 weeks for individuals who have insomnia, but, again, there are no long-term studies. Data on other antidepressants (eg, amitriptyline and mirtazepine) in individuals who have chronic insomnia are lacking. All antidepressants have potentially significant adverse effects, raising concerns about the risk-benefit ratio. The dose-response relationship needs to be established for all these agents [27].

A number of other sedating medications, such as antipsychotics, have been used in the treatment of insomnia. Considering the significant risks of these agents, their use in the treatment of chronic insomnia cannot be recommended, especially in the elderly [27].

Nonprescription medications

Melatonin

Melatonin was discovered in 1958 as a hypnotic, and is a naturally occurring neurohormone primarily produced by pineal gland. Its secretion is timed by the oscillation of the endogenous circadian rhythm. Melatonin acts on suprachiasmatic nucleus causing adjustment in the timing of the circadian rhythm. A systemic review of treatment of insomnia in older adults of six double blind randomized control trials has been evaluated. In these trials polysomnography or wrist actigraphy were measured. Five of the trials showed improvement in sleep latency or sleep efficacy when compared with placebo. One study showed improved sleep in patients who were using benzodiazepines in the past. The sample size of these studies varied from 10 to 26 subjects. This review did not find any causal relationship between low melatonin levels and insomnia in the elderly. There was also no change in subjective sleep improvement and deep sleep was not increased [34]. In a double-blind, placebo-control trial, 15 subjects aged 50 years and older were monitored with polysomnography and were given three melatonin doses (0.1 mg, 0.3 mg, and 3.0 mg) orally 30 minutes before bedtime for a week. At all doses, sleep efficacy in the middle and later third of the night was improved, but there was no change in deep sleep or any other objective parameters [35].

Singer and colleagues [36] studied the efficacy of melatonin on insomnia in Alzheimer's patients, in a multicenter, randomized, placebo-controlled trial. Subjects with Alzheimer's disease and nighttime sleep disturbance were randomly assigned to one of three treatment groups: placebo, 2.5-mg slow-release melatonin, or 10-mg melatonin. This study was conducted in private homes and long-term care facilities and included 157 subjects who were treated for 2 months. No statistically significant differences in objective sleep measures were seen between baseline and treatment periods for any of the three groups.

Valerian

Valerian is a perennial plant native to Asia and Europe and naturalized in North America. Preparation of valerian marketed as dietary supplements are made from its root, rhizomes, and stolons. Valerian had been used as an herbal medicine by ancient Greece and Rome, but its therapeutic effect was first described by Hippocrates. Galen prescribed valerian for insomnia in the second century. There is no agreement on the uniform mechanism of valerian pharmacologic activity. The mechanism of action could be through GABA agonistic activity [37], or possible effect through adenosine and 5HT-5a receptors [38,39].

Few studies have examined the effect of valerian on sleep in older adults. The first trial by Kamm-Khol and colleagues [40] studied 80 subjects who were in geriatric hospitals and received valerian or placebo for 2 weeks. Sleep improvement was assessments by two validated questionnaires and a sleep rating scale. There was improvement in sleep latency and duration; however, it did not include studies in objective measures of sleep, relying solely on questionnaires.

Shultz and colleagues [41] studied 14 older female subjects who were poor sleepers; sleep outcome was measured with polysomnography after 8 days of treatment with valerian. Valerian improved deep sleep significantly, and decreased stage 1 sleep compared with placebo, suggesting overall improved sleep quality, but this study was limited by a small sample size.

Antihistamine

Antihistamines, such as diphenhydramine, may be used for their sedating effects. They are associated with daytime drowsiness, sedation, dizziness, dry mucous membranes, blurring of vision, urinary retention, constipation, and other anticholinergic effects, and cognitive impairment [7,42].

Medication with strong antihistamine properties should be avoided because of potential side effects in older adults. There is no data to support that antihistamines either prolong sleep or improve sleep [43].

Side effects

Older adults are more likely to be chronic hypnotic users [44] and are more vulnerable to the hazards associated with hypnotics, in part because of slower drug absorption and elimination. Because older adults consume more medications in general there is a heightened risk of polypharmacy complications [45]. Serious potential side effects of hypnotic use in the elderly are more closely related to long half-life benzodiazepines. Examples include increased automobile accidents [46] and a higher rate of falls producing hip fracture [47] and femur fracture [48]. Allen and colleagues [49] reported that zolpidem was considered as a risk for falls in one study among older adults.

Summary

From the review of the literature, benzodiazepines, when use to treat insomnia, could result in unwanted side effects such as falls, confusions, hang over, or fracture of the hip and femur. These medications should be avoided if at all possible. The newer nonbenzodiazepines, although less studied in older adult at this stage, appear to have fewer side effects and are well tolerated. There is no ideal agent available for the treatment of insomnia in older adults; more trials are needed to include frail and robust older adults and compare the currently available prescription and nonprescription medications. More research is needed to evaluate the long-term effects of treatment and the most appropriate management strategy for older adults with chronic insomnia.

References

[1] Walsh JK, Engelhardt CL. Trends in the pharmacologic treatment of insomnia. J Clin Psychiatry 1992;53:10–8.
[2] Ohayon MM, Caulet M, Priest RG, et al. Psychotropic medication consumption patterns in the UK general population. J Clin Epidemiol 1998;51:273–83.
[3] Maggi S, Langlois JA, Minicuci N, et al. Sleep complaints in community-dwelling older persons: prevalence, associated factors, and reported causes. J Am Geriatr Soc 1998;46: 161–8.
[4] Ozminkowski RJ, Wang S, Walsh JK. The direct and indirect costs of untreated insomnia in adults in the United States. Sleep 2007;30(3):263–73.
[5] Weitzel KW, Wickman JM, Augustin SG, et al. Zaleplon: a pyrazolopyrimidine sedative-hypnotic agent for the treatment of insomnia. Clin Ther 2000;22:1254–67.
[6] Morin CM. Measuring outcomes in randomized clinical trials of insomnia treatments. Sleep Med Rev 2003;7(3):263–79.
[7] Woodward M. Hypnosedatives in the elderly. A guide to appropriate use. CNS Drugs 1999; 11:263–79.
[8] Grunstein R. Insomnia: diagnosis and management. Aust Fam Physician 2002;31:1–6.
[9] Montgomery P. Treatments for sleep problems in elderly people. Br Med J 2002;325: 1049–51.
[10] Shochat T, Loredo J, Ancoli-Israel S. Sleep disorders in the elderly. Curr Treat Options Neurol 2001;3:19–36.
[11] Vgontzas AN, Kales A, Bixler EO, et al. Temazepam 7.5 mg: effects on sleep in elderly insomniacs. Eur J Clin Pharmacol 1994;46(3):209–13.
[12] Glass J, Lanctot KL, Herrmann N, et al. Sedative hypnotics in older people with insomnia: meta-analysis of risks and benefits. BMJ 2005;331:1169–76.
[13] The risk for injury in the elderly may vary by benzodiazepine, independent of half-life [review]. ACP J Club 2005;143(1):24.
[14] Sedative-hypnotics increase adverse effects more than they improve sleep quality in older persons with insomnia [review]. ACP J Club 2006;145(1):14.

[15] Lavoisy J, Zivkovic B, Benavides J, et al. Contribution of Zolpidem in the management of sleep disorders. Encephale 1992;18:379–92.

[16] Shaw SH, Curson H, Coquelin JP. A double-blind, comparative study of zolpidem and placebo in the treatment of insomnia in elderly psychiatric in-patients [erratum appears in]. J Int Med Res 1992;20(2):150–61, 1992.

[17] Holm KJ, Goa KL. Zolpidem. An update of its pharmacology, therapeutic efficacy and tolerability in the treatment of insomnia. Drugs 2000;59:865–89.

[18] Kupfer DJ, Reynolds CF. Management of insomnia. N Engl J Med 1997;336:341–6.

[19] Hedner J, Yaeche R, Emilien G, et al. Zaleplon shortens subjective sleep latency and improves subjective sleep quality in elderly patients with insomnia. The Zaleplon Clinical Investigator Study Group. Int J Geriatr Psychiatry 2000;15:704–12.

[20] Ancoli-Israel S, Walsh JK, Mangano RM, et al. Zaleplon, a novel nonbenzodiazepine hypnotic, effectively treats insomnia in elderly patients without causing rebound effects. Prim Care Companion J Clin Psychiatry 1999;1:114–20.

[21] Ancoli-Israel S, Richardson GS, Mangano RM. Long-term use of sedative hypnotics in older patients with insomnia. Sleep Med 2005;6:107–13.

[22] McCall WV, Erman M, Krystal AD, et al. A polysomnography study of eszopiclone in elderly patients with insomnia. Curr Med Res Opin 2006;22:1633–42.

[23] Scharf M, Erman M, Rosenberg R, et al. A 2-week efficacy and safety study of eszopiclone in elderly patients with primary insomnia. Sleep 2005;28:720–7.

[24] Zammit GK, McNabb LJ, Caron J, et al. Efficacy and safety of eszopiclone across 6 weeks of treatment for primary insomnia. Curr Med Res Opin 2004;20:1979–91.

[25] Krystal AD, Walsh JK, Eugene, et al. Sustained efficacy of eszopiclone over 6 months of nightly treatment: results of a randomized, double-blind, placebo controlled study in adults with chronic insomnia. Sleep 2003;26:793–9.

[26] Najib J. Eszopiclone, a nonbenzodiazepine sedative-hypnotic agent for the treatment of transient and chronic insomnia. Clin Ther 2006;28(4):491–516.

[27] NIH State of the Science Conference Statement on insomnia. Manifestations and management of chronic insomnia in adults. June 13–15, 2005. Sleep 2005;28:1049–58.

[28] Roth T, Stubbs C, Walsh JK. Ramelteon (TAK-375), a selective MT1/MT2 receptor agonist reduces latency to persistent sleep in a model of transient insomnia related to a novel environment. Sleep 2005;28:303–7.

[29] Roth T, Seiden D, Zee P, et al. Phase III trial of Ramelteon for the treatment of chronic insomnia in elderly patients. J Am Geriatr Soc 2005;53:S25.

[30] Dolder C, Nelson M, McKinsey J. Use of non-benzodiazepine hypnotics in the elderly: are all agents the same? CNS Drugs 2007;21(5):389–405.

[31] Brian KT. Management of chronic insomnia in elderly persons. Am J Geriatr Pharmacother 2006;4(2):168–92.

[32] Mendelson WB. A review of the evidence for the efficacy and safety of trazadone in insomnia. J Clin Psychiatry 2005;66(4):469–76.

[33] James SP, Mendelson WB. The use of trazodone as a hypnotic: a critical review. J Clin Psychiatry 2004;65(6):752–5.

[34] Old Rikkert MG, Rigaud AS. Melatonin in elderly patients with insomnia. A systemic review. Z Gerontol Geriatr 2001;34:491–7.

[35] Zhdanova IV, Wurtman RJ, Regan MM, et al. Melatonin treatment for age-related insomnia. J Clin Endocrinol Metab 2001;86(10):4727–30.

[36] Singer C, Tractenberg RE, Kaye J, et al. A multicenter, placebo-controlled trial of melatonin for sleep disturbance in Alzheimer's disease. Sleep 2003;26(7):893–901.

[37] Santos MS, Ferreira F, Cunha AP, et al. Synaptosomal GABA release as influenced by valerian root extract-involvement of the GABA carrier. Arch Int Pharmacodyn Ther 1994;327:220–31.

[38] Dietz BM, Mahady GB, Pauli GF, et al. Valerian extract and valerenic acid are partial agonist of the 5 HT [5a] receptors in vitro. Brain Res 2005;138:191–7.

[39] Schumacher B, Scholle S, Holzl J, et al. Lignans isolated from valerian: identification and characterization of a new olivil derivative with partial agonistic activity at A [1] adenosine receptors. J Nat Prod 2002;65:1479–85.

[40] Kamm-Khol AV, Jansen W, Brockmann P. Moderne baldriantherapie gegen vervose strorungen im semium [Modern valerian therapy for nervous disorder in old age]. Med Welt 1984; 35:1450–4 [German].

[41] Shultz H, Stolz C, Muller J. The effect of Valerian extract on sleep polygraphy in poor sleepers: a pilot study. Pharmacopsychiatry 1995;27:147–51.

[42] Neubauer DN. Sleep problems in the elderly. Am Fam Physician 1999;59:2551–8.

[43] Ancoli-Israel S. Sleep problems in older adults putting myths to bed. Geriatrics 1997;52: 20–30.

[44] Morgan K, Clarke D. Longitudinal trends in late-life insomnia: implications for prescribing. Age Ageing 1997;26:179–84.

[45] Lebowitz BD, Niederehe G. Concepts and issues in mental health and aging. In: Birren JE, Sloane RB, Cohen GD, editors. Handbook of mental health and aging. 2nd edition. San Diego (CA): Academic Press; 1992. p. 3–26.

[46] Neutel CI. Risk of traffic accident injury after a prescription for a benzodiazepine. Ann Epidemiol 1995;5:239–44.

[47] Ray WA, Griffin MR, Downey W. Benzodiazepines of long and short elimination half-life and the risk of hip fracture. JAMA 1989;262:3303–7.

[48] Herings RMC, Stricker BHC, de Boer A, et al. Benzodiazepines and the risk of falling leading to femur fractures: dosage more important than elimination half-life. Arch Intern Med 1995;155:1801–7.

[49] Allan H, Bentue-Ferrer D, Polard E, et al. Postural instability and consequent falls and hip fractures associated with use of hypnotics in the elderly: a comparative review. Drugs Aging 2005;22(9):749–65.

ELSEVIER
SAUNDERS

CLINICS IN
GERIATRIC
MEDICINE

Clin Geriatr Med 24 (2008) 107–119

Nonpharmacologic Therapy for Insomnia in the Elderly

Seema Joshi, MD

*Bettendorf Internal Medicine and Geriatrics,
4480 Utica Ridge Road, Suite 160, Bettendorf, IA 52722, USA*

Nonpharmacologic therapy for insomnia in the elderly

Sleep changes over the life span. Approximately 50% of older Americans report chronic difficulties with their sleep [1]. Complaints of insomnia are more common in women and their prevalence increases with advancing age [2]. Objective evidence for these complaints has been demonstrated by polysomnography. Aging is associated with several well-described changes in sleep architecture [3]. The most significant change is a phase advance of the normal circadian cycle. Thus, the elderly tend to have an earlier onset of sleep that is accompanied by an earlier morning wake signal. The elderly often go to bed early and report being early risers [4]. A recent meta-analysis revealed that with age, percentages of stage 1 and 2 sleep increased, whereas the percentage of rapid eye movement (REM) and slow-wave sleep decreased. Thus, more of the night was spent in the lighter stages of sleep [5].

Older adults have a decrease in their ability to maintain sleep; however, the absolute need for sleep does not decrease with age. Sleep becomes more fragmented in older adults, resulting in a decrease in sleep efficiency (amount of time spent in bed asleep) which continues to decrease after the age of 60. Though sleep is shorter in duration, shallower, and more fragmented in the elderly, poor sleep is not an inevitable consequence of aging [6].

Insomnia is frequently multifactorial. Sleep complaints in the older adult may be comorbid with chronic medical and psychiatric conditions. Several factors have been implicated in the development of insomnia in the older adult. These include:

- Comorbid medical and neurologic conditions
- Medications

E-mail address: seemajoshi@hotmail.com

0749-0690/08/$ - see front matter © 2008 Elsevier Inc. All rights reserved.
doi:10.1016/j.cger.2007.08.005   *geriatric.theclinics.com*

- Psychologic and behavioral factors
- Environmental and social factors
- Primary sleep disorders, such as sleep apnea, restless legs syndrome, and REM behavior disorder

The above factors, either alone or in combination, can compromise an individual's sleep quality [7,8]. Older adults with more than three medical conditions are more likely to complain of insomnia and excessive daytime sleepiness [9]. Medications may cause or contribute to insomnia.

Sleep disturbances are associated with significant morbidity and mortality. Studies have revealed that chronic insomnia is associated with a higher risk of death [10,11]. Insomnia is also thought to be a risk factor for depression, anxiety, substance abuse, and suicide [12]. Sleep disorders may also have a negative impact on health-related quality of life by increasing the risk of accidents, malaise, and chronic fatigue [13]. Insomnia may be associated with decreased memory and concentration, and impaired performance on psychomotor tests. Chronic insomnia independently predicts incident cognitive decline in older men [14,15].

Nonpharmacologic and pharmacologic approaches are effective for the short-term management of insomnia in late life; however, current evidence suggests that sleep improvements are better sustained over time with behavioral treatment [16–19]. This article provides an overview of nonpharmacologic approach for the treatment of insomnia.

Nonpharmacologic management of insomnia

Management of insomnia that is secondary to medical illness should start with treatment of the primary disease process. If the individual's history suggests a primary sleep disorder or a sleep-related movement disorder, the patient may need nocturnal polysomnographic recordings to establish the diagnosis. Nondrug treatment of insomnia is quite effective and underutilized by health care professionals. Nondrug treatments involve behavioral, cognitive, and physiologic interventions. Common methods of cognitive behavior therapy (CBT) for insomnia include:

- Relaxation
- Stimulus control
- Sleep restriction
- Cognitive interventions or therapy
- Sleep education and sleep hygiene
- Light therapy
- Chronotherapy

Numerous controlled studies have shown improvement in the quality and quantity of sleep in primary insomnia. CBT is safe and effective, and its various components can be used alone or in combination for the treatment of insomnia [20]. Relaxation therapy is designed to reduce psychologic and physiologic stress. The association between sleep and the bedroom environment is reinforced in stimulus control therapy. Sleep restriction involves restriction of the amount of time spent in bed to that equivalent to the amount of nighttime sleeping. Sleep hygiene involves identifying behaviors detrimental to sleep and encouraging those that promote sleep. The different modalities of CBT are discussed in further detail in the following sections.

Relaxation therapy and imagery

Thoughts can be detrimental to sleep and anxiety may cause sleep onset insomnia. Relaxation training originally used to alleviate anxiety is used for the treatment of sleep onset insomnia. Several techniques have been used in the treatment of insomnia. These modalities include [21–23]:

- Progressive muscle relaxation
- Autogenic training—this relaxation technique focuses on increasing blood flow to the legs and arms. Induction of sensations of warmth and heaviness are used to promote somatic relaxation.
- Imagery—pleasant imagery can be used along with relaxation to improve sleep.

Individuals must practice the chosen technique at least twice a day. It may require several weeks of practice before the skill is acquired. This technique must not be used initially to induce sleep.

In a study by Lichstein and Johnson [24] of older women with insomnia, the treatment effect with relaxation therapy was dependent on the medication status (hypnotic versus nonhypnotic) of the insomniac. There was substantial sleep improvement among nonhypnotically medicated insomniacs and substantial sleep medication reduction (47%) was seen among hypnotically medicated insomniacs.

In another study, community dwelling older adults with insomnia were randomized to relaxation, sleep compression, and placebo desensitization. The study involved collection of data using questionnaires and polysomnography at baseline, posttreatment, and 1-year follow-up. The study showed an improvement in self-reported sleep, but objective sleep was unchanged. However, results partially supported the conclusion that individuals with daytime impairment respond best to treatments that extend sleep, as in relaxation, and individuals with low daytime impairment respond best to treatments that consolidate sleep, as in sleep compression [25].

Stimulus control

To cope with being awake during the night, many individuals with chronic insomnia engage in behaviors in the bedroom that contribute to insomnia. These may include worrying, reading, and watching television, among other behaviors. In a study of subjects with sleep onset insomnia, there was an improvement in sleep in 70% of the subjects when they consistently followed the practice of having only 10 minutes to fall asleep (20 minutes in the elderly) [26]. The purpose of stimulus control is to break the association between maladaptive behaviors and arousal. Instructions to patients for stimulus control include:

1. Go to bed only if you feel sleepy
2. Avoid activities in the bedroom that keep you awake, other than sex
3. Sleep only in your bedroom
4. Leave the bedroom when awake
5. Return to the bedroom only when sleepy
6. Arise at the same time each morning, regardless of the amount of sleep obtained that night
7. Avoid daytime napping

Stimulus control treatment instructions have been modified slightly for older adults. These modifications include increasing the estimated sleep-onset latency to 15 to 20 minutes and the permissibility of one short nap [27]. In a controlled comparative investigation of psychologic treatment of patients with chronic insomnia, subjects were randomly allocated to progressive relaxation, stimulus control, paradoxical intention, placebo, or no treatment. Active treatments were associated with significant improvement in sleep. However, gains varied depending on the nature of treatment. Stimulus control was associated with improved sleep pattern, whereas relaxation affected perception of sleep quality. All improvements were maintained at 17-month follow-up [28]. The efficacy of stimulus control therapy has been shown by several controlled studies to be efficacious in the treatment of both sleep-onset and sleep-maintenance insomnia [28–31].

Sleep restriction therapy

Sleep restriction therapy has been shown to be an effective treatment for common forms of chronic insomnia. In a study by Spielman and colleagues [32], sleep restriction in subjects with chronic insomnia increased total sleep time ($P<0.05$) as well as improved sleep latency, total wake time, sleep efficiency, and subjective assessment of insomnia (all $P<0.0001$). Improvement remained significant for all sleep parameters on follow up at 36 weeks posttreatment. The efficacy of sleep restriction alone or in combination with other modalities has been shown in controlled trials [33,34].

Sleep restriction therapy causes sleep deprivation, resulting in an increase in sleep drive. Before initiation of sleep restriction therapy the individual is required to keep a sleep log for 2 weeks. This helps in estimating the average sleep time versus time spent in bed. The allowed sleep time is the average subjective sleep time, but is never less than 5 hours. The time in bed is adjusted by 15-minute increments or decrements, depending on the sleep efficiency. Sleep efficiency is defined as the average sleep time or time in bed times 100%. If sleep efficiency is greater than 90%, the time in bed is increased by 15 minutes, and if it is less than 85%, the time is decreased by 15 minutes. Approximately 25% of patients benefit from this treatment [35].

Cognitive interventions

Research shows that CBT can be used successfully in the treatment of insomnia [18,36]. Although formal cognitive therapy is increasingly used as part of CBT, it has not been evaluated as a single therapy for insomnia. CBT addresses maladaptive behaviors, dysfunctional cognition, and misconceptions related to insomnia. It helps the patient identify beliefs that are counterproductive. Cognitive therapy is designed to identify dysfunctional cognitions and reframe them into more adaptive substitutes to short-circuit the self-fulfilling nature of this vicious cycle. Treatment targets may include unrealistic expectations, faulty causal attributions, and amplification of the consequences of insomnia. It challenges behaviors incompatible with sleep [37].

In a randomized controlled trial of 63 adults with chronic sleep-onset insomnia, CBT was found to be superior to pharmacologic management with zolpidem [18]. Current evidence suggests that CBT may be as effective as prescription medications for brief treatment of chronic insomnia. Additionally, the beneficial effects of CBT are sustained beyond the treatment period. There is no evidence that CBT is associated with adverse effects [16–19]. However, the relative efficacy of nonpharmacologic therapies remains to be established. In a meta-analysis of 59 trials sleep hygiene measures alone did not show efficacy. Also, when used on their own, sleep restriction and stimulus control therapies were more effective than relaxation therapy [16]. The 2005 National Institutes of Health State-of-the-Science Conference on Insomnia concludes that CBT is as effective as prescription medications for the treatment of chronic insomnia [38]. However, clinical benefits of CBT may not be seen until a few weeks after initiation of treatment [39].

Sleep education and hygiene

Sleep hygiene measure alone are not sufficient for the treatment of insomnia; however, they may be useful when used in conjunction with other modalities. Sleep hygiene addresses health practices, habits, and environmental factors that impact sleep. Physicians need to educate patients regarding sleep and its disorders. It is important to emphasize that simple lifestyle changes can help in the treatment of insomnia. Box 1 lists some of the sleep-related practices and habits that may interfere with sleep. It is important to foster good sleeping habits.

Box 1. Health Practices and habits that may impair sleep

- Frequent daytime napping and nodding
- Sleeping extra hours during the weekend
- Spending too much time in bed
- Insufficient daytime activities
- Late evening exercises
- Insufficient morning light exposure
- Excess caffeine
- Evening alcohol consumption
- Smoking in the evening
- Late heavy dinner
- Watching television or engaging in other stimulating activities
- Anxiety and anticipation of poor sleep
- Clock watching
- Environmental factors, such as the room being too warm, too noisy, or too bright

---

Several factors may contribute to insomnia in the elderly. Behavioral factors particularly in the elderly may include alcohol, caffeine, nicotine intake, and exercising too close to bedtime. An unfavorable sleep environment, such as too much light or noise, may be disruptive to sleep. Excessive daytime napping, lack of exercise, and inadequate light exposure during the day can contribute to insomnia. Many older individuals may be taking over-the-counter or herbal medications with stimulant properties. Patients may not volunteer this information unless specifically asked, and simple measures may help with improved sleep in the elderly.

Light therapy

The circadian system is responsible for the 24-hour sleep and wake cycle. In human beings the endogenous circadian rhythm is slightly longer than 24 hours. This predisposes the endogenous rhythm to gradually shift later in time. Genetic determinants for the circadian rhythm have been identified in animals and human beings [40–43]. Circadian rhythm disorders can cause insomnia because of a lack of synchronization between an individual's internal clock and the external schedule. Sleep disorders seen with circadian rhythm disorders include delayed sleep phase disorder, when sleep time is delayed in relation to the desired clock time, and advanced sleep phase disorder, when the patient goes to sleep in the early evening and wakes up earlier than desired in the morning.

Exposure to bright light can stabilize or shift the endogenous rhythm [44,45]. Early morning light exposure is used to treat patients with a delayed sleep phase. Bright light exposure is administered in the morning as close to the patient's scheduled arising time as possible. Light therapy counters the inherent shift toward a later phase and can be useful in maintaining a 24-hour circadian period [46]. Evening bright light exposure has been used to treat patients with advance sleep phase disorders and tends to delay the circadian sleep phase [47].

The endogenous circadian rhythm responds to the shorter wavelengths of the visible spectrum. The peak sensitivity is at a wavelength of about 470 nm, which corresponds to blue color. Light therapy can be achieved with natural sunlight or artificial light using a light box. Light therapy with artificial light is done using 10,000 lux for 30 to 40 minutes upon awakening. Evening light exposure must be reduced to achieve the desired results in individuals with delayed phase sleep disorders. Blue-blocking sunglasses may be worn to counter the phase-delaying effect of evening light exposure. Response is usually seen in 2 to 3 weeks and maintenance of response frequently requires indefinite treatment [48–53]. Similarly, in individuals with advanced phase disorder a light box should be used in the evenings. The use of sun glasses that block blue light in the morning may be helpful [47].

Chronotherapy

Chronotherapy involves a progressive delay of bedtime, usually 2 to 3 hours per night, until the desired earlier bedtime is achieved. This treatment modality has shown success in individuals with delayed phase disorder, which is relatively common in adolescents and young adults [54]. It is not a modality of choice for the treatment of insomnia in the elderly.

Nonpharmacologic treatment of insomnia in long-term care setting

Sleep is fragmented among nursing home residents, who often stay in bed awake for prolonged periods of time [55,56]. A study by Alessi and Schnelle [57] showed that nursing home residents slept only 58% of the time while in bed. Also, studies done by Ancoli-Israel and colleagues on nursing home residents, have revealed that residents at the nursing home are seldom awake or asleep for a full hour at any point during the day or night [58,59].

Multiple factors contribute to abnormal sleep-wake patterns in nursing home residents. Certain potentially reversible behavioral and environmental factors may contribute to sleep problems in the long-term care setting. These potentially modifiable factors include limited sunlight exposure, large amounts of time spent in bed, lack of physical activity, a disruptive night-time environment, and other factors that lead to poor sleep hygiene [60,61]. A randomized, controlled trial of nonpharmacologic intervention

Box 2. Practice parameters for nonpharmacologic treatment of chronic insomnia [66]

Recommendations according to type of insomnia
- Psychologic and behavioral interventions are effective and recommended in the treatment of chronic primary insomnia.
- Psychologic and behavioral interventions are effective and recommended in the treatment of secondary insomnia.
- Stimulus control therapy is effective and recommended therapy in the treatment of chronic insomnia.
- Relaxation training is effective and recommended therapy in the treatment of chronic insomnia.
- Sleep restriction is effective and recommended therapy in the treatment of chronic insomnia.
- Cognitive behavior therapy, with or without relaxation therapy, is effective and recommended therapy in the treatment of chronic insomnia.
- Multicomponent therapy (without cognitive therapy) is effective and recommended therapy in the treatment of chronic insomnia.
- Paradoxical intention is effective and recommended therapy in the treatment of chronic insomnia.
- Biofeedback is effective and recommended therapy in the treatment of chronic insomnia.
- Insufficient evidence was available for sleep hygiene education to be an option as a single therapy. Whether this therapy is effective when added to other specific approaches could not be determined from the available data.
- Insufficient evidence was available for imagery training to be an option as a single therapy. Whether this therapy is effective when added to other specific approaches could not be determined from the available data.
- Insufficient evidence was available for cognitive therapy to be recommended as a single therapy.
- Insufficient evidence was available to recommend one single therapy over another, or to recommend single therapy versus a combination of psychologic and behavioral interventions.

Recommendations relevant to specific patient groups
- Psychologic and behavioral interventions are effective and recommended in the treatment of insomnia in older adults.
- Psychologic and behavioral interventions are effective and recommended in the treatment of insomnia among chronic hypnotic users.

Areas for future research
- Studies are needed to evaluate the effectiveness of psychologic and behavioral treatments, not only in reducing insomnia symptoms but also in improving measures of clinical significance, such as daytime function, quality of life, and morbidity. This issue has also been raised in the 2005 National Institutes of Health State of the Science Conference Statement regarding chronic insomnia.
- In studies of secondary insomnia, research is needed to determine whether targeting sleep symptoms leads to an improvement in sleep, regardless of whether or not there is improvement in the underlying condition.
- Further research is needed comparing the effectiveness of different single psychologic and behavioral therapies for insomnia.
- Further research is also needed to address whether there is an added benefit of providing a combination of psychologic and behavioral therapies over a single therapy, and to identify patient groups where combination or single therapy is most appropriate.
- Studies are needed that compare pharmacologic and psychologic or behavioral treatments of insomnia, as well as combined therapies in terms of their short and long-term effectiveness, risk, benefits, costs, and patient satisfaction.

to improve abnormal sleep-wake patterns in nursing home residents reported decreased daytime sleeping and increased participation in social and physical activities and social conversation [62]. Another randomized controlled trial of nonpharmacologic intervention among nursing home residents, suggested that these interventions may effectively improve the robustness of rest and activity rhythms [63]. However, a multicomponent, nonpharmacologic intervention trial by Ouslander and colleagues [64] was unable to demonstrate any effect on nighttime sleep.

The treatment of insomnia in the nursing population can be challenging; however, simple measures, such as limiting daytime naps to 1 hour in the early afternoon, avoiding stimulating medications, foods and beverages, providing a bright daytime environment, quiet, and dark night environment may be helpful [65].

Summary of evidence

The evidence regarding the efficacy of nonpharmacologic treatments for insomnia has been reviewed by a task force appointed by the American

Academy of Sleep Medicine and published in the journal Sleep in 2006 [66]. This report reviewed 37 clinical trials to develop practice parameters for nonpharmacologic management of chronic insomnia. A summary of the American Academy of Sleep Medicine Practice Parameters for nonpharmacologic treatment of chronic insomnia is included in Box 2.

The task force concluded that nonpharmacologic therapies produce reliable and durable changes in several sleep parameters of chronic insomnia sufferers. Data also indicate that between 70% and 80% of patients treated with nonpharmacologic interventions benefit from treatment. Nondrug treatment of insomnia is likely to reduce the symptoms of sleep onset latency or wake time after sleep onset. It is also associated with an increase in sleep duration by a modest 30 minutes, and improved sleep quality and patient's satisfaction with sleep patterns. Sleep improvements achieved with these behavioral interventions are sustained for at least 6 months after treatment completion [39].

An evaluation of behavioral treatments for insomnia in the older adult population indicated that sleep hygiene, stimulus control, progressive relaxation alone or in combination were effective in improving the sleep diary assessed awakenings, naptime, and feeling refreshed upon awakening. Stimulus control appeared to be most effective in improving sleep in the posttherapy period. In addition, behavioral treatments were found to be effective in improving perception of sleep in older adults with insomnia [67].

Outcome research is needed to examine the effectiveness of nondrug treatment of insomnia in the elderly when it is implemented in clinical settings by nonsleep specialists, and in insomnia patients with medical or psychiatric comorbidity.

Summary

Insomnia is prevalent in the elderly. It is associated with an increased morbidity and mortality. Older adults have a decrease in their ability to maintain sleep; however, the absolute need for sleep does not decrease with age. Poor sleep is not an inevitable consequence of aging. Older adults often have multiple comorbid conditions, are on multiple medications, and are therefore predisposed to adverse drug reactions. Evidence suggests that nonpharmacologic treatments are effective and well suited for the clinical management of insomnia in the elderly. Non pharmacologic modalities may be used alone or in combination with pharmacologic therapy for effective treatment of insomnia in the elderly.

References

[1] Foley DJ, Monjan AA, Brown SL, et al. Sleep complaints among elderly persons: an epidemiologic study of three communities. Sleep 1995;18:425–32.

[2] Ohayon MM. Epidemiology of insomnia: what we know and what we still need to learn. Sleep Med Rev 2002;6:97–111.

[3] Bliwise DL. Review: sleep in normal aging and dementia. Sleep 1993;16:40–81.

[4] Wolkove N, Elkholy O, Baltzan M, et al. Sleep and aging: 1. Sleep disorders commonly found in older people. CMAJ 2007;176(9):1299–304.

[5] Ohayon MM, Carskadon MA, Guilleminault C, et al. Meta-analysis of quantitative sleep parameters from childhood to old age in healthy individuals: developing normative sleep values across the human lifespan. Sleep 2004;27:1255–73.

[6] Rajput V, Bromley SM. Chronic Insomnia: A Practical Review. American Family Physician. 1999;60(5).

[7] Vitiello MV, Moe KE, Prinz PN. Sleep complaints co-segregate with illness older adults: clinical research informed by and informing epidemiological studies of sleep. J Psychosom Res 2002;53:555–9.

[8] Vitiello MV. Normal versus pathological sleep changes in aging humans. In: Kuna ST, Suratt PM, Remmers JE, editors. Sleep and respiration in aging adults. New York: Elsevier; 1991. p. 71–6.

[9] Foley D, Ancoli-Israel S, Britz P, et al. Sleep disturbances and chronic disease in older adults: results of the 2003 National Sleep Foundation Sleep in America Survey. J Psychosom Res 2004;56:497–502.

[10] Dew MA, Hoch CC, Buysse DJ, et al. Healthy older adults' sleep predicts all-cause mortality at 4 to 19 years of follow-up. Psychosom Med 2003;65:63–73.

[11] Manabe K, Matsui T, Yamaya M, et al. Sleep patterns and mortality among elderly patients in a geriatric hospital. Gerontology 2000;46:318–22.

[12] Taylor DJ, Lichstein KL, Durrence HH. Insomnia as a health risk factor. Behav Sleep Med 2003;1:227–47.

[13] Schubert CR, Cruickshanks KJ, Dalton DS, et al. Prevalence of sleep problems and quality of life in an older population. Sleep 2002;25:889–93.

[14] Grunstein R. Insomnia. Diagnosis and management. Aust Fam Physician 2002;31:1–6.

[15] Cricco M, Simonsick EM, Foley DJ. The impact of insomnia on cognitive functioning in older adults. J Am Geriatr Soc 2001;49:1185–9.

[16] Morin CM, Culbert JP, Schwartz SM. Nonpharmacological interventions for insomnia: a meta-analysis of treatment efficacy. Am J Psychiatry 1994;151:1172–80.

[17] Morin CM, Colecchi C, Stone J, et al. Behavioral and pharmacological therapies for late-life insomnia: a randomized controlled trial. JAMA 1999;281:991–9.

[18] Jacobs GD, Pace-Schott EF, Stickgold R, et al. Cognitive behavior therapy and pharmacotherapy for insomnia. Arch Intern Med 2004;164:1888–96.

[19] Smith MT, Perlis ML, Park A, et al. Comparative meta-analysis of pharmacotherapy and behavior therapy for persistent insomnia. Am J Psychiatry 2002;159:5–11.

[20] Harvey AG, Tang NKY. Cognitive behaviour therapy for primary insomnia: can we rest yet? Sleep Med Rev 2003;7:237–62.

[21] Nicassio P, Bootzin R. A comparison of progressive relaxation and autogenic training as treatment for insomnia. J Abnorm Psychol 1974;83:253–60.

[22] Borkovec TD, Grayson JB, O'Brien GT, et al. Relaxation treatment of pseudoinsomnia and idiopathic insomnia: an electroencephalographic evaluation. J Appl Behav Anal 1979;12:37–54.

[23] Woolfolk RL, Carr-Kaffashan L, McNulty TF. Meditation training as a treatment for insomnia. Behav Ther 1976;7:359–65.

[24] Lichstein KL, Johnson RS. Relaxation for insomnia and hypnotic medication use in older women. Psychol Aging 1993;8:103–11.

[25] Lichstein KL, Riedel BW, Wilson NM, et al. Relaxation and sleep compression for late-life insomnia: a placebo-controlled trial. J Consult Clin Psychol 2001;69:227–39.

[26] Bootzin R. Stimulus control treatment for insomnia. Proceedings of the 80th annual convention of the American Psychological Association 1972;7:395–6.

[27] Bootzin RR, Epstein D. Stimulus control. In: Lichstein KL, Morin CM, editors. Treatment of late-life insomnia. Thousand Oaks (CA): Sage Publications, Inc; 2000. p. 167–84.
[28] Espie CA, Lindsay WR, Brooks DN, et al. A controlled comparative investigation of psychological treatments for chronic sleep-onset insomnia. Behav Res Ther 1989;27:79–88.
[29] Morin CM, Azrin NH. Stimulus control and imagery training in treating sleep-maintenance insomnia. J Consult Clin Psychol 1987;55:260–2.
[30] Riedel B, Lichstein KL, Peterson BA, et al. comparison of the efficacy of stimulus control for medicated and nonmedicated insomniacs. Behav Modif 1998;22:3–28.
[31] Morin CM, Azrin NH. Behavioral and cognitive treatments of geriatric insomnia. J Consult Clin Psychol 1988;56:748–53.
[32] Spielman AJ, Saskin P, Thorpy MJ. Treatment of chronic insomnia by restriction of time in bed. Sleep 1987;10:45–56.
[33] Friedman L, Bliwise DL, Yesavage JA, et al. A preliminary study comparing sleep restriction and relaxation treatments for insomnia in older adults. J Gerontol 1991;46:1–8.
[34] Friedman L, Benson K, Noda A, et al. An actigraphic comparison of sleep restriction and sleep hygiene treatments for insomnia in older adults. J Geriatr Psychiatry Neurol 2000;13:17–27.
[35] Lacks P, Morin CM. Recent advances in the assessment and treatment of insomnia. J Consult Clin Psychol 1993;60:586–94.
[36] Edinger JD, Wohlgemuth WK, Radtke RA, et al. Cognitive behavioral therapy for treatment of chronic primary insomnia: a randomized controlled trial. JAMA 2001;285:1856–64.
[37] Morin CM, Espie CA. Insomnia: a clinical guide to assessment and treatment. New York: Kluwer Academics/Plenum Publishers; 2003.
[38] NIH State of the Science Conference Statement on Insomnia. Manifestations and management of chronic insomnia in adults. Sleep 2005;28:1049–58.
[39] Morin CM, Hauri PJ, Espie CA, et al. Nonpharmacologic treatment of chronic insomnia. An American Academy of Sleep Medicine review. Sleep 1999;22:1134–56.
[40] Wager-Smith K, Kay SA. Circadian rhythm genetics: from flies to mice to humans. Nat Genet 2000;26:23–7.
[41] Klei L, Reitz P, Miller M, et al. Heritability of morningness-eveningness and self-report sleep measures in a family-based sample of 521 Hutterites. Chronobiol Int 2005;22:1041–54.
[42] Dijk DJ, Czeisler CA. Contribution of the circadian pacemaker and the sleep homeostat to sleep propensity, sleep structure, electroencephalographic slow waves, and sleep spindle activity in humans. J Neurosci 1995;15:3526–38.
[43] Czeisler CA, Duffy JF, Shanabar TL, et al. Stability, precision, and near-24-hour period of the human circadian pacemaker. Science 1999;284:2177–81.
[44] Wagner DR. Disorders of the circadian sleep-wake cycle. Neurol Clin 1996;14:651–70.
[45] Richardson GS, Malin HV. Circadian rhythm sleep disorders: Pathophysiology and treatment. J Clin Neurophysiol 1996;13:17.
[46] Rosenthal NE, Joseph-Vanderpool JR, Levendosky AA, et al. Phase-shifting effects of bright morning light as treatment for delayed sleep phase syndrome. Sleep 1990;13:354–61.
[47] Campbell SS, Dawson D, Anderson MW. Alleviation of sleep maintenance insomnia with timed exposure to bright light. J Am Geriatr Soc 1993;41:829–36.
[48] Thapan K, Arendt J, Skene DJ. An action spectrum for melatonin suppression: evidence for a novel non-rod, non-cone photoreceptor system in humans. J Phys 2001;535:261–7.
[49] Lockley SW, Brainard GC, Czeisler CA. High sensitivity of the human circadian melatonin rhythm to resetting by short wavelength light. J Clin Endocrinol Metab 2003;88:4502–5.
[50] Brainard GC, Hanifin JP, Greeson JM, et al. Action spectrum for melatonin regulation in humans: evidence for a novel circadian photoreceptor. J Neurosci 2001;21:6405–12.
[51] Chesson AL Jr, Littner M, Davila D, et al. Practice parameters for the use of light therapy in the treatment of sleep disorders. Standards of Practice Committee, American Academy of Sleep Medicine. Sleep 1999;22:641–60.
[52] Mahowald MW, Chokroverty S, Kader G, Schenck CH. Sleep disorders. Continuum. A Program of the American Academy of Neurology, 1997. p. 56.

[53] Sasseville A, Paquet N, Sevigny J, et al. Blue blocker glasses impede the capacity of bright light to suppress melatonin production. J Pineal Res 2006;41:73–8.

[54] Czeisler CA, Richardson GS, Coleman RM, et al. Chronotherapy: Resetting the circadian clocks of patients with delayed sleep phase syndrome. Sleep 1981;4:1–21.

[55] Van Haitsma K, Lawton MP, Kleban MH, et al. Methodological aspects of the study of streams of behavior in elders with dementing illness. Alzheimer Dis Assoc Disord 1997;11: 228–38.

[56] Pat-Horenczyk R, Klauber MR, Shochat T, et al. Hourly profiles of sleep and wakefulness in severely versus mild-moderately demented nursing home patients. Aging Clin Exp Res 1998; 10:308–15.

[57] Alessi CA, Schnelle JF. Approach to sleep disorders in the nursing home setting. Sleep Med Rev 2000;4:45–56.

[58] Ancoli-Israel S, Parker L, Sinaee R, et al. Sleep fragmentation in patients from a nursing home. J Gerontol 1989;44(1):M18–21.

[59] Ancoli-Israel S, Klauber MR, Jones DW, et al. Variations in circadian rhythms of activity, sleep and light exposure related to dementia in nursing home patients. Sleep 1997;20:18–23.

[60] Schnelle JF, Cruise PA, Alessi CA, et al. Sleep hygiene in physically dependent nursing home residents. Sleep 1998;21:515–23.

[61] Schnelle JF, Ouslander JG, Simmons SF, et al. The nighttime environment, incontinence care, and sleep disruption in nursing homes. J Am Geriatr Soc 1993;41:910–4.

[62] Alessi CA, Martin JL, Webber AP, et al. Randomized, Controlled Trial of a Nonpharmacological Intervention to Improve Abnormal Sleep/Wake Patterns in Nursing Home Residents. J Am Geriatr Soc 2005;53:803–10.

[63] Martin JL, Marler MR, Harker JO, et al. A Multicomponent Nonpharmacological Intervention Improves Activity Rhythm Among Nursing Home Residents with Disrupted Sleep/Wake Patterns. Journ of Geron: Medical Sciences 2007;62A(1):67–72.

[64] Ouslander JG, Cornell BR, Bliwise DL, et al. A Non Pharmacological Intervention to Improve Sleep in Nursing Home Patients: Results of Controlled Trial. JAGS 2006;54:38–47.

[65] Ancoli-Israel S, Jones DW, McGuinn P, et al. Sleep disorders. In: Morris J, Lipshitz J, Murphy K, et al, editors. Quality care for the nursing home. St. Louis (MO): Mosby Lifeline; 1997. p. 64–73.

[66] Morgenthaler T, Kramer M, Alessi C, et al. American Academy of Sleep Medicine. Practice parameters for the psychological and behavioral treatment of insomnia: an update. An American Academy of Sleep Medicine report. Sleep 2006;29(11):1415–9.

[67] Engle-Friedman M, Bootzin RR, Hazelwood L, et al. An evaluation of behavioral treatments for insomnia in the older adult. Journ of Clin psych 1992;48(1):77–90.

ELSEVIER
SAUNDERS

Clin Geriatr Med 24 (2008) 121–138

CLINICS IN
GERIATRIC
MEDICINE

Complementary and Alternative Medicine for Sleep Disturbances in Older Adults

Nalaka S. Gooneratne, MD, MSc, ABSM

Division of Geriatric Medicine, Center for Sleep and Respiratory Neurobiology, University of Pennsylvania School of Medicine, 3615 Chestnut Street, Philadelphia, PA 19104, USA

Complementary and alternative medicines (CAM) have a long history of use for the treatment of sleep disorders. In the second century AD, for example, the prominent ancient Greek physician Galen (Claudius Galenus) prescribed valerian for insomnia [1]. CAM therapies are defined by the National Center for Complementary and Alternative Medicine (NCCAM) as "a group of diverse medical and health care systems, practices, and products that are not presently considered to be part of conventional medicine" [2]. While the terms are often used synonymously, a more accurate statement is the NCCAM definition that complementary medicines are "used together with conventional medicine," while alternative medicines are "used in place of conventional medicine" (Fig. 1) [2]. Inherent in this definition of CAM is a concept of change: what is considered to be a CAM therapy today may become a conventional form of treatment in the future. An example of this would be the growth of clinical patient support groups or the use of some forms of cognitive-behavioral therapy as mainstream medical treatments [2].

There exist several hundred different forms of CAM therapy. The classification method used by NCCAM consists of five broad domains (See Fig. 1): (1) Alternative medical systems that are based on a set of theories and practices that have generally developed apart from conventional medicine. These include acupuncture, Ayurveda, or homeopathy. (2) Biologically based practices, which consist of compounds often found in nature, such as herbal products. (3) Mind-body medicine, which uses systems of thought

Funding from grant numbers NCCAM R01 AT001521, NIA K23 AG01021, UL1 RR024134 (University of Pennsylvania CTSA).

E-mail address: ngoonera@mail.med.upenn.edu

doi:10.1016/j.cger.2007.08.002 *geriatric.theclinics.com*

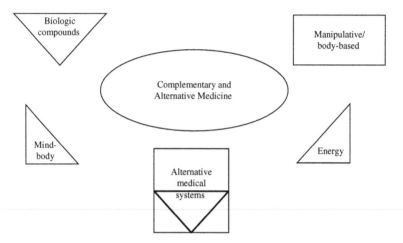

Fig. 1. Diagram of complementary and alternative medicine (CAM) subtypes. Alternative medical systems may often contain elements from other forms of CAM.

that can affect bodily functions. This is a broad category that can include meditation, Tai Chi, yoga, and biofeedback. (4) Manipulative and body-based practices that rely on movement of select parts of the body. An example would be massage-based therapies. (5) Energy medicine that emphasizes the use of energy fields, including bio-electromagnetic based therapies [2].

Many CAM therapies, in particular the biologically based practices and some forms of alternative medical systems, are regulated under the Dietary Supplemental and Education Act of 1994. According to these guidelines, these compounds are not required to undergo purity, safety, or efficacy testing. Standardization of compounds across different research studies is thus not always consistent, and some products may not contain the ingredients they advertise. Furthermore, under these guidelines, these products cannot claim treatment effects for specific disease processes in their marketing or advertising.

This article focuses on CAM therapies for sleep disorders in older adults. Because there are a large number of CAM therapies, the discussion is limited to the therapies that are most widely used, and for which an adequate body of scientific data exists upon which to base conclusions. Since there is a relative paucity of literature for certain modalities, the article also reviews studies on sleep treatment in younger subjects where appropriate. Several reviews exist of CAM therapy to which the reader is referred for more information about specific modalities [3–14]. The major categories that are discussed in this article include the following (Fig. 2): alternative medical systems, such as acupuncture and Ayurveda; biologic compounds, such as melatonin and valerian; mind-body therapies, such as meditation, yoga, Tai Chi; and manipulation, such as massage.

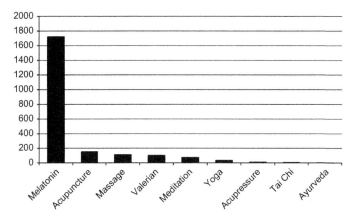

Fig. 2. Number of publications of different types of CAM for sleep based on Medline search.

CAM usage by older adults

A recent telephone survey of 1,559 people over the age of 50, conducted by the American Association of Retired Persons and NCCAM, noted that 54% of persons aged 65 or older had used a CAM therapy or practice [15]. The 30% response rate, fairly typical for telephone surveys that do not offer financial compensation, may have overestimated CAM use because users may be more likely to respond than nonusers. Nevertheless, the overall prevalence of use is quite high.

When considering factors that influenced CAM use, individuals with a higher income or more years of college education were more likely to use CAM [15]. Much of the information obtained by older adults regarding CAM therapies came from family or friends (22%), publications (14%), or radio/TV/internet (20%). Only 31% of CAM users had discussed CAM with their physician and only 12% obtained information about CAM from their physicians [15]. This highlights the need for physicians to inquire about CAM and help educate their patients regarding CAM. Furthermore, asking about CAM use can help a physician to minimize the risk of poly-pharmacy: 75% of those who had taken an herbal or dietary product during their lifetime were also taking one or more prescription medications [15].

The majority of patients with insomnia also have comorbidities: only 4.1% of patients with insomnia did not have a comorbidity [16]. In older adults, many of whom are taking multiple medications, the potential inter-actions between CAM products and conventional medicine are important to consider. Unfortunately, there is a relative paucity of literature dealing with this topic (Fig. 3).

When considering the use of CAM for insomnia in particular, a recent analysis of the National Health Interview Survey dataset (74.3% response rate) by Pearson and colleagues [16] revealed that 4.5% of adults (over age 18, noninstitutionalized) used some form of CAM for their insomnia

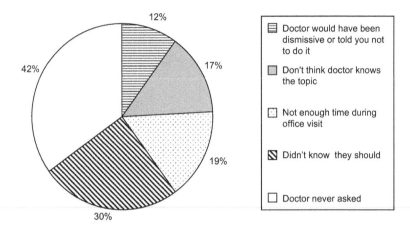

Fig. 3. Reasons cited for not having discussed CAM with their physician. (*Data from* American Association of Retired Persons, National Center for Complimentary and Alternative Medicine. Complementary and alternative medicine: what people 50 and over are using and discussing with their physicians. Washington, D.C.: AARP; 2007.)

or trouble sleeping in the past year. Other sedative prescription drugs, by comparison, are used by approximately 5% to 10% of adults (age over 16–18 years) with insomnia [17,18]. Another interesting observation was that the prevalence of CAM use in those with insomnia tended to decrease with age (Fig. 4). The most commonly used CAM modalities in adults were biologically based therapies (64.8% of adult CAM users) and mind-body

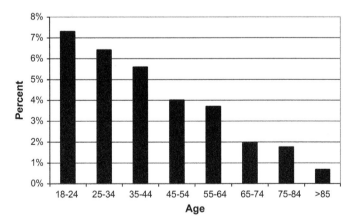

Fig. 4. Prevalence of CAM use by age group. (*Adapted from* Pearson et al. "Insomnia, trouble sleeping, and complementary and alternative medicine: Analysis of the 2002 national health interview survey data," Arch Inter Med, 2006;166(16):1775–82; with permission.)

therapies (39.1% of adult CAM users); those with comorbidities tended to prefer biologically based therapies [16].

Melatonin

Melatonin is one of the most thoroughly studied CAM biologic compounds used for sleep. It is a hormone produced by the pineal gland that is postulated to play a significant role in regulating the sleep-wake cycle [19]. It has low daytime circulating levels and elevated nocturnal levels that coincide with the sleep phase [20]. Melatonin has the ability to influence the timing of the circadian sleep-wake cycle, as has been demonstrated by work in subjects with a free-running circadian rhythm [21]. It may also have sedative effects, possibly via direct inhibition of the suprachiasmatic nucleus via a feedback loop [22,23]. Melatonin injected into other brain regions, such as the medial preoptic area, can induce sleep as well [24].

Numerous studies have shown decreased melatonin levels in the elderly relative to subjects under age 30 [25–27]. This may in part occur because of declines in the number of pinealocytes [28], or neuronal degeneration of the suprachiasmatic nucleus and resultant circadian desynchrony [29]. The presence of insomnia itself is also independently associated with serum melatonin deficiency in some studies [30,31] but not in others [29,32–34]. Melatonin deficiency is caused by three potential factors: medications, age-related changes, and melatonin suppression from comorbid medical condition. Melatonin is profoundly decreased by a variety of medications commonly used by the elderly, including beta-blockers [35] and nonsteroidal anti-inflammatory drugs [36]. The extent of melatonin suppression may be more profound in the elderly than in younger subjects [37]. In addition to medications, a variety of primary conditions, such as chronic pain [38], myocardial infarction [39], and ischemic stroke [40] are strongly associated with decreased melatonin levels. This melatonin deficiency is particularly problematic in the elderly, as animal studies have shown decreased levels of the melatonin 1a receptor with aging [41].

These findings have led to a strong interest in using exogenous melatonin to treat chronic primary insomnia in older adults. Doses have ranged from 0.1 mg to 0.3 mg (which results in physiologic melatonin levels) to 5 mg to 10 mg (pharmacologic melatonin levels). Initial studies showed evidence of a benefit [42], including reduced sleep latency in patients with cognitive impairment [43]; however, these studies relied on wrist-activity assessment of sleep-wake. Other wrist-activity studies have been negative, however [44]. In the largest study to date that uses objective measures, Singer and colleagues [45] studied 157 older adults with Alzheimer's Disease and randomized them into three groups: placebo, melatonin 2.5-mg sustained release, and melatonin 10 mg. There was no statistically significant benefit on objective parameters (wrist-activity monitoring) with melatonin therapy; this was the primary study measure. Caregivers did note improvement in sleep (as assessed using a sleep diary) for patients using the 2.5-mg sustained-release formulation relative to placebo or the 10-mg immediate release formulation; however, there was no significant difference in the subjective sleep disturbance index scores amongst the study arms.

More rigorous studies relying on polysomnography (which is often required by the Food and Drug Administration for sedative-hypnotics to show efficacy) have also been conducted. Some studies have shown a benefit [46,47], while others did not demonstrate significant improvements in sleep patterns [48,49].

Recently, a large meta-analysis was conducted of melatonin therapy for sleep [50]. The meta-analysis suggested that melatonin had a clinically insignificant benefit for primary insomnia in older adults: there was a 7.8-minute improvement in sleep latency, but no overall improvement in sleep efficiency. Patients with delayed sleep phase syndrome did show a larger, clinically significant benefit of 38.8 minutes. No benefit was noted for secondary insomnia.

Attempts have also been made to target specific subgroups of patients by their melatonin profile. For example, one study by Hughes and colleagues [48] found no overall benefit, but noted that the most prominent improvement occurred in subjects who had a short duration of endogenous melatonin secretion. Of note, this study had an unusual treatment regimen in which all subjects were awoken 4.5 hours after the initial melatonin dose to take a middle-of-the-night dose. One actigraphy-based study in subjects with low melatonin levels noted improved sleep [51]; however, only the first 6 hours of sleep were analyzed in this study. Another self-report study found evidence of benefit [52]; however the interpretation of these results is limited by the study design, which consisted of a nonrandomized placebo and melatonin paradigm. Alternative forms of melatonin have also been tested, including transbuccal melatonin, with no significant benefit in elderly subjects with insomnia [49].

In general, melatonin is well tolerated in the dose range of 0.1 mg to 10 mg with few reported adverse events [53–55]. One particular concern in the elderly, however, is that of daytime sleepiness [56]. No clinical trials of melatonin in the elderly have measured objective markers of daytime sleepiness. However, one study in younger subjects using objective measures of performance suggests that the sedative effects of melatonin persist even up to 7 hours after ingestion [57], and another study noted "tiredness at rising" in four (out of eleven) subjects treated with melatonin [58]. Thus, while melatonin has the potential to improve sleep efficiency and thereby result in decreased daytime sleepiness, its use may directly lead to daytime sleepiness if the melatonin is taken very late in the evening. It is also possible that melatonin doses of 3 mg to 5 mg may lead to increased sleep disruption, as has been noted in 4 of 16 younger subjects given melatonin in a temporal isolation study [59]. Despite these concerns, Jean-Louis and colleagues [43], in their previously mentioned study of melatonin 6 mg in cognitively-impaired subjects, noted improved memory recall and concentration, and no increased subjective fatigue. In addition, melatonin is less likely to lead to dependence and abuse, as can occur with other sedative-hypnotics, as it does not cause euphoria [60].

A large body of work has been done examining melatonin's effects on other organ systems in regards to its safety profile. These findings are summarized below.

Cardiovascular effects

Human studies using doses, such as melatonin 5 mg, have observed that melatonin may impair the antihypertensive efficacy of calcium channel blockers to a mild degree. In subjects on nifedipine who were treated with melatonin, there was a mean increase in systolic blood pressure of 6.5 mm Hg, and in diastolic blood pressure of 4.9 mm Hg [61]. Human studies show mild reduction in blood pressure with physiologic doses of melatonin [62].

Immune system effects

Melatonin may have immunomodulatory effects, although no clear consensus exists in this regard as to overall safety [63]. Some studies have suggested a proinflammatory role in conditions, such as autoimmune arthritis [64,65], while others have found melatonin to be protective against the development of autoimmune disorders, such as type I diabetes mellitus [66], and experimental models of inflammation, such as carrageenan [67]. There has also been one case report regarding the development of autoimmune hepatitis in a patient taking melatonin [68]. Of note, the melatonin formulation taken by the patient may have contained unknown additives [69].

Other effects

In one study of bipolar disorder, the use of melatonin 10 mg for 3 months has been associated with suppression of endogenous melatonin and the development of an unentrained (free-running) sleep-wake cycle, after melatonin withdrawal in two of five subjects [70]; research in nonbipolar disorder subjects has shown no suppression of endogenous melatonin, however (A. Lewy, personal communication). Melatonin may increase the severity of sleep apnea, as noted in one study that documented mild to moderate increases in sleep apnea in some subjects taking melatonin [71]. Melatonin may affect follicle stimulating hormone (FSH), luteotropic hormone (LH), and thyroid hormones; however, this has not been found to have significant clinical effects in older adults [72,73]. Other side effects noted with melatonin include headache and pruritis in less than 10% of subjects [74].

To examine these concerns, several studies have evaluated the safety of melatonin. One study, using 10 mg over a 1 month period, documented no evidence of adverse events in younger subjects [54]. An open-label study of 22 older subjects (mean age 60.1 years) with 3 mg of melatonin for 6 months found no significant changes in endocrine and routine chemistry and liver function analysis, including FSH, LH, and thyroid stimulating hormone [53]. Another study administered 1 mg for 2 months in elderly subjects, with no reported side effects [51]. In an extended open-label study of 2-mg of melatonin nightly for 6 months, elderly subjects had decreased estra-diol levels, and increased insulin-like growth factor-1 (IGF-1) and dehydro-piandrosterone sulfate levels, but no adverse clinical events occurred [75].

There have also been two large reviews of melatonin that have been pub-lished recently (2004). The first review was conducted by the Institute of Medicine/National Academies [76]. This 70-page article observed that the only cardiovascular adverse event noted with melatonin, from approxi-mately 60 clinical studies (including both young, middle-aged, and elderly subjects), was an increase in blood pressure of approximately 6.5 mm Hg in hypertensive patients on calcium channel blockers, as mentioned earlier. A second large review of melatonin was recently published by the Agency for Health care Research and Quality [50]. The article concluded that ad-verse "effects were not significant compared with placebo." They also con-cluded that melatonin is a "relatively safe substance" in the short term.

Overall, the current evidence suggests that melatonin has a clear role in the management of circadian sleep disorders, such as delayed sleep phase syndrome. The evidence is more equivocal for primary or secondary insom-nia, or for the treatment of insomnia in patients with cognitive impairment. It may be that in certain subgroups, such as patients with low melatonin levels or abnormal timing of their melatonin cycle, exogenous melatonin may have a beneficial role; however, more work is needed in this area. For-tunately, melatonin appears to have a relatively benign side effect profile.

Valerian

The plant species Valeriana, in particular *Valeriana officinalis* and to a lesser extent *Valeriana edulis*, is the source of the ingredients in valerian. These ingredients can be divided into the following categories: valepotriates, sesquiterpenes (volatile oil components which account for valerian's un-pleasant odor), and amino acids (such as γ-aminobutyric acid or GABA, and glutamine) [77]. Putative sites of action of valerian include the GABA receptor [78], binding at A(1) adenosine receptors [79] or, as more recently noted, the 5-HT-5a receptor [80].

The extraction and preparation method can influence the relative concen-trations of each of the valerian components in a given formulation, thus one issue with clinical studies of valerian compounds is that while each study may use "valerian," the specific components may differ. Standardization and purity of biologically based compounds can be a concern, and this ap-plies also to valerian compounds. A recent report by ConsumerLab.com noted that 4 of 17 valerian products had no detectable valerian content, four had half the amount listed, two had lead contamination, and one had cadmium contamination [81].

Valerian has been studied in several randomized, placebo-controlled studies, in doses ranging from 400 mg to 900 mg [5,6]. One study, using both subjective and objective (polysomnography and actigraphy) measures in 18 subjects without sleep problems, noted that while subjective measures improved, objective measures showed small, clinical and statistically insignificant improvements [82]. Another actigraphy-based study observed a statistically significant improvement in sleep latency (from 15.8 plus or minus 5.8 minutes, to 9.0 plus or minus 3.9 minutes, $P < 0.01$) in subjects with insomnia; however, higher doses of 900 mg were associated with morning sleepiness [83]. Polysomnography-based research has also shown that a prolonged (2-week) course of treatment was associated with reductions in sleep latency, but no overall change in sleep efficiency [84]. Leathwood and colleagues [85] conducted a study in which subgroup analysis included older adult poor sleepers. They noted that 63% reported subjective improvement with valerian; however, 43% also noted improvement with placebo and there was thus no statistically significant difference. Valerian has also been used as a tool to assist with weaning patients from benzodiazepines, with some limited success. Sleep quality improved and wakefulness after sleep onset decreased; however, there was an increased sleep latency [86]. Comparisons with benzodiazepines, such as oxazepam, have also been performed and have found that valerian was as effective as oxazepam in improving sleep; however, it was not a placebo-controlled study and relied on subjective self-report [87]. Valerian has also been used in combination with other agents, such as hops. This valerian-hops combination resulted in a reduced self-reported sleep latency of 5.6 minutes ($P = 0.079$) relative to placebo, and all other subjective and polysomnographic measures were similar.

Studies specifically targeting older adults with insomnia have also been conducted using objective measures. A randomized, placebo-controlled study of 14 subjects noted that total sleep time and slow-wave sleep improved with valerian [88]. The valerian group, however, had significantly worse baseline sleep parameters, thus making it difficult to determine if these results represent a true effect of valerian or a regression toward the mean phenomenon. A later study using a one night dosing paradigm found no significant benefit of valerian relative to placebo [89].

In general, valerian has been found to be safe with minimal side effects in the published literature. Rare side effects that have been reported include gastrointestinal upset, contact allergies, headache, restless sleep, and mydriasis [90]. In comparison with placebo, adverse events occurred at a similar rate, and there were no rebound insomnia or withdrawal effects with valerian [91]. Valerian has been considered as a possible treatment for sleep disruption in comorbid medical states, such as cancer [92] and rheumatoid arthritis [93]; however, because of uncertainty regarding polypharmacy and metabolism, it is not recommended for use in critically ill patients [94]. Valepotriates may also alkylate DNA, and can thus have theoretical cytotoxic and carcinogenic potential [77]. Because valerian may act on GABA receptors, valerian may potentiate the sedative effects of other central nervous system depressants [95]. Research examining the daytime "hangover" cognitive effects found no difference between placebo and valerian [91,96]. There is also a case report of valerian withdrawal symptoms which were characterized by delirium in a patient who had been using 0.5 grams to 2 grams per dose up to five times daily for several years; symptoms improved with benzodiazepine therapy [97].

In summary, valerian has been studied in several randomized, placebo-controlled trials, including several studies in older adults. There appears to be evidence of a mild subjective improvement in sleep with valerian, especially when used for 2 weeks or more. However, the objective testing has had less consistent results with little or no improvement noted. Some, but not all, studies have observed increased slow-wave sleep, which could be an important finding if validated in additional work. Methodologic limitations, nonstandardized formulations, and the small sample size of the existing literature (which creates a higher likelihood of type-2 errors), suggests that future larger studies are needed once a well-characterized and standardized form of valerian is developed.

Manipulative and body-based practices

The manipulative and body-based practices encompass a broad range of therapies that involve hands-on interventions. The majority of the published literature on massage therapy are for sleep disorders in infants and children. Studies in adult populations are limited and tend to focus on subjects with comorbid medical conditions. One study examined the use of aromatherapy massage for hospice patients using self-report measures of sleep. This randomized, placebo-controlled study noted no benefits in quality of life or pain control; however, there were statistically significant improvements in sleep and depression [98]. Another randomized study, comparing therapeutic massage and relaxation tapes in the management of stress, noted that while patients expressed a preference for massage, both modalities showed improvements in sleep, with no significant benefit of one over the other [99]. Combination therapies using massage have also suggested a benefit, although these often have not included a placebo arm [100]. Polysomnography studies of massage have also been conducted: Richards [101] conducted a randomized trial of a massage intervention compared with placebo, and observed a 1-hour increase in sleep time for the massage therapy group. Massage therapy has also been used for fibromyalgia, where it has been found to increase sleep time and reduce pain levels [102,103].

Another form of manipulative therapy is acupressure, which is a noninvasive technique that involves stimulation of meridian or acupoints on the body using finger pressing movements. It can be administered by nursing staff or by family members of a patient. Acupressure has been studied in a randomized design in institutionalized older adults [104]. This study noted statistically significant improvements in both the Pittsburgh Sleep Quality Index (primary outcome measure) and number of nocturnal awakenings in the acupressure group relative to the two placebo arms (sham acupressure and conversation). This group has also studied acupressure in end-stage renal patients using a similar design, and also observed evidence of statistically significant improvements in self-reported sleep quality, sleep latency, and sleep efficiency [105]. Another study has replicated these findings [106]. Agitated behavior in patients with dementia has also been treated with acupressure, with one study noting reductions in the Cohen-Mansfield Agitation Inventory score, and other metrics of agitation in subjects during the acupressure arm relative to the control arm [107].

Another form of acupressure is auricular therapy, which involves applying pressure to acupoints either via the fingertips, medicinal seeds, or magnets [108,109]. Suen and colleagues [109] conducted a 3-week randomized, single-blind placebo-controlled study using wrist-activity monitoring to provide an objective assessment of sleep parameters between magnetic auricular acupressure and two controls. They observed statistically significant improvements in sleep latency and sleep efficiency, with an overall increase of approximately 35 minutes in the total sleep time. Adverse effects were not discussed in their article; however, auricular therapy is generally considered safe. A 6-month follow-up of this cohort was also conducted and found that insomnia symptoms remained ameliorated in the treatment group relative to the control groups [108].

The results of these studies are very intriguing. However, this work needs to be replicated in additional studies amongst more diverse cohorts before it can be routinely recommended for the management of insomnia.

Acupuncture

Acupuncture, which is considered in the category of alternative medical systems, also acts on meridian points to influence health [9]. The majority of studies using acupuncture have relied on subjective measures or have not had a placebo control, thus making interpretation of study findings difficult [9]. Few studies have examined the effects of acupuncture in insomnia using polysomnography [110,111]. While both demonstrated evidence of improved sleep, one was a pilot study that was not placebo-controlled [110]. This study also demonstrated increases in nocturnal melatonin secretion and reductions in stress and anxiety scores, compared with pretreatment levels.

Acupuncture has also been examined as a treatment modality for sleep disruption because of other conditions, including insomnia post stroke [112] and postmenopausal symptoms [113,114]. Other sleep disorders that have been treated with acupuncture include fibromyalgia [115,116] and sleep apnea [117,118].

Meditation

While there are several forms of meditation, one of the most commonly studied for insomnia is mindfulness meditation. Stress reduction may be one of the mechanisms by which meditation can exert a beneficial effect on sleep and most of the studies that have demonstrated improved sleep during meditation therapy have been conducted as stress reduction studies. In this regard, it can be used as part of a cognitive therapy approach. In addition to stress reduction, there may also be differences in slow-wave sleep as a result of meditation [119]. Meditation therapy has also been used in cancer patients and found to help improve sleep in two studies [120,121].

Yoga

Yoga is a multicomponent practice that consists of physical activity associated with specific postures, breathing exercises, and a specific philosophic attitude toward life. It has been shown to reduce anxiety levels and physiologic arousal. A randomized, parallel group study conducted over a 6-month treatment period compared yoga (60 minute session 6 days a week, with a 15 minute evening session), Ayurvedic therapy, and wait-list control in 69 older adults [122]. Self-reported sleep measures were assessed and demonstrated a 1-hour increase in total sleep time relative to pretreatment that was significantly higher than changes in the wait-list or Ayurveda groups. When studied in other populations, such as lymphoma patients, yoga was found to improve subjective sleep parameters when compared with a wait-list control group [123,124].

Tai Chi

Tai Chi is a low- to moderate-intensity Chinese exercise that includes a meditational component. A study of the effects of Tai Chi (consisting of three 60 minutes sessions for 24 weeks) in 118 older adults, in comparison to low-impact exercise, noted that Tai Chi improved self-reported sleep duration by 48 minutes [125]. General health-related quality of life and daytime sleepiness levels also improved. No injuries were reported in either group. Of note, 33% of subjects withdrew from the study (no significant difference between the Tai Chi and exercise groups). These findings are very interesting and if replicated by additional research using objective measures, could add to the CAM treatment options for insomnia.

Summary

This article presents the main CAM therapies for sleep disorders in older adults on which adequate published evidence exists. By far, the largest body of work has been done with melatonin, which has been found to have a benefit in the treatment of circadian sleep disorders, with more equivocal results for primary or secondary insomnia. Valerian has also been found to improve sleep in some studies, but variability in extraction and formulation remains an issue. Other therapies that have shown promise in a limited number of studies include acupuncture, acupressure, yoga, meditation, and Tai Chi. The findings from these studies need to be replicated in additional work at different sites in more diverse patient groups that would help to validate the early findings. Most of the CAM therapies discussed have benign side effect profiles from the limited body of data currently available. Thus, they hold the potential to significantly benefit sleep in older adults, a population most at risk for polypharmacy and altered drug metabolism. Increased emphasis on objective measures, more rigorous study design (parallel arm placebo-controlled designs) and larger study sample sizes are crucial next steps for the field.

References

[1] Natural Standard Research Collaboration. Valerian (Valeriana officinalis L.). [internet] Oct 1, 2006. Available at: http://www.nlm.nih.gov/medlineplus/druginfo/natural/patient-valerian.html. Accessed May 20, 2007.

[2] National Center for Complementary and Alternative Medicine. What Is CAM? NCCAM Publication No. D347. [internet] February 2007. Available at: http://nccam.nih.gov/health/whatiscam/. Accessed June 1, 2007.

[3] Meoli AL, Rosen CL, Kristo D, et al. Non-Pharmacologic Treatments for Insomnia. J Clin Sleep Med 2005;1:173–87.

[4] Shimazaki M, Martin JL. Do herbal agents have a place in the treatment of sleep problems in long-term care? J Am Med Dir Assoc 2007;8(4):248–52.

[5] Bent S, Padula A, Moore D, et al. Valerian for sleep: a systematic review and meta-analysis. Am J Med 2006;119(12):1005–12.

[6] Stevinson C, Ernst E. Valerian for insomnia: a systematic review of randomized clinical trials. Sleep Med 2000;1(2):91–9.

[7] Wheatley D. Medicinal plants for insomnia: a review of their pharmacology, efficacy and tolerability. J Psychopharmacol 2005;19(4):414–21.

[8] Management of insomnia: a place for traditional herbal remedies. Prescrire Int 2005;14(77):104–7.

[9] Sok SR, Erlen JA, Kim KB. Effects of acupuncture therapy on insomnia. J Adv Nurs 2003;44(4):375–84.

[10] Larzelere MM, Wiseman P. Anxiety, depression, and insomnia. Prim Care 2002;29(2):339–60, vii.

[11] Crofford LJ, Appleton BE. Complementary and alternative therapies for fibromyalgia. Curr Rheumatol Rep 2001;3(2):147–56.

[12] Gyllenhaal C, Merritt SL, Peterson SD, et al. Efficacy and safety of herbal stimulants and sedatives in sleep disorders. Sleep Med Rev 2000;4(3):229–51.

[13] Vallbona C, Richards T. Evolution of magnetic therapy from alternative to traditional medicine. Phys Med Rehabil Clin N Am 1999;10(3):729–54.

[14] Lin Y. Acupuncture treatment for insomnia and acupuncture analgesia. Psychiatry Clin Neurosci 1995;49(2):119–20.

[15] American Association of Retired Persons, National Center for Complementary and Alternative Medicine. Complementary and Alternative Medicine: what People 50 and Over Are Using and Discussing with Their Physicians. Washington, D.C.: AARP; 2007.

[16] Pearson NJ, Johnson LL, Nahin RL. Insomnia, trouble sleeping, and complementary and alternative medicine: analysis of the 2002 national health interview survey data. Arch Intern Med 2006;166(16):1775–82.

[17] Hatoum HT, Kania CM, Kong SX, et al. Prevalence of insomnia: a survey of the enrollees at five managed care organizations. Am J Manag Care 1998;4(1):79–86.

[18] Stewart R, Besset A, Bebbington P, et al. Insomnia comorbidity and impact and hypnotic use by age group in a national survey population aged 16 to 74 years. Sleep 2006;29(11): 1391–7.

[19] Zhdanova IV. Melatonin as a hypnotic: pro. Sleep Med Rev 2005;9(1):51–65.

[20] Brzezinksi A. Melatonin in Humans. N Engl J Med 1997;336(3):186.

[21] Sack RL, Brandes RW, Kendall AR, et al. Entrainment of free-running circadian rhythms by melatonin in blind people. N Engl J Med 2000;343(15):1070–7.

[22] Dubocovitch M. Melatonin receptors: are there multiple subtypes? Trends Pharmacol Sci 1995;16:50–6.

[23] Liu C, Weaver DR, Jin X, et al. Molecular dissection of two distinct actions of melatonin on the suprachiasmatic circadian clock. Neuron 1997;19(1):91–102.

[24] Mendelson WB. Melatonin microinjection into the medial preoptic area increases sleep in the rat. Life Sci 2002;71(17):2067–70.

[25] Zhou JN, Liu RY, Van Heerikhuize J, et al. Alterations in the circadian rhythm of salivary melatonin begin during middle-age. J Pineal Res 2003;34(1):11–6.

[26] Touitou Y, Fevre M, Lagoguey M, et al. Age- and mental health-related circadian rhythms of plasma levels of melatonin, prolactin, luteinizing hormone and follicle-stimulating hormone in man. J Endocrinol 1981;91(3):467–75.

[27] Sharma M, Palacios-Bois J, Schwartz G, et al. Circadian rhythms of melatonin and cortisol in aging. Biol Psychiatry 1989;25(3):305–19.

[28] Humbert W, Pevet P. Calcium content and concretions of pineal glands of young and old rats. A scanning and X-ray microanalytical study. Cell Tissue Res 1991;263(3): 593–6.

[29] Kripke DF, Elliot JA, Youngstedt SD, et al. Melatonin: marvel or marker? Ann Med 1998; 30(1):81–7.

[30] Riemann D, Klein T, Rodenbeck A, et al. Nocturnal cortisol and melatonin secretion in primary insomnia. Psychiatry Res 2002;113(1–2):17–27.

[31] Hajak G, Rodenbeck A, Staedt J, et al. Nocturnal plasma melatonin levels in patients suffering from chronic primary insomnia. J Pineal Res 1995;19(3):116–22.

[32] Youngstedt SD, Kripke DF, Elliott JA, et al. Circadian abnormalities in older adults. J Pineal Res Oct 2001;31(3):264–72.

[33] Lushington K, Dawson D, Kennaway DJ, et al. The relationship between 6-sulphatoxyme-latonin and polysomnographic sleep in good sleeping controls and wake maintenance insomniacs, aged 55–80 years. J Sleep Res 1999;8(1):57–64.

[34] Baskett JJ, Wood PC, Broad JB, et al. Melatonin in older people with age-related sleep maintenance problems: a comparison with age matched normal sleepers. Sleep 2001; 24(4):418–24.

[35] Van Den Heuvel CJ, Reid KJ, Dawson D. Effect of atenolol on nocturnal sleep and temperature in young men: reversal by pharmacological doses of melatonin. Physiol Behav 1997;61(6):795–802.

[36] Murphy PJ, Myers BL, Badia P. Nonsteroidal anti-inflammatory drugs alter body temperature and suppress melatonin in humans. Physiol Behav 1996;59(1):133–9.

[37] Surrall K, Smith JA, Bird H, et al. Effect of ibuprofen and indomethacin on human plasma melatonin. J Pharm Pharmacol 1987;39(10):840–3.

[38] Almay BG, von Knorring L, Wetterberg L. Melatonin in serum and urine in patients with idiopathic pain syndromes. Psychiatry Res 1987;22(3):179–91.

[39] Brugger P, Marktl W, Herold M. Impaired nocturnal secretion of melatonin in coronary heart disease. Lancet 1995;345(8962):1408.

[40] Fiorina P, Lattuada G, Silvestrini C, et al. Disruption of nocturnal melatonin rhythm and immunological involvement in ischaemic stroke patients. Scand J Immunol 1999;50(2): 228–31.

[41] Richardson G, Tate B. Hormonal and pharmacological manipulation of the circadian clock: recent developments and future strategies. Sleep 2000;23(Suppl 3):S77–85.

[42] Garfinkel D, Laudon M, Nof D, et al. Improvement of sleep quality in elderly people by controlled-release melatonin. Lancet 1995;346(8974):541–4.

[43] Jean-Louis G, von Gizycki H, Zizi F. Melatonin effects on sleep, mood, and cognition in elderly with mild cognitive impairment. J Pineal Res 1998;25(3):177–83.

[44] Baskett JJ, Broad JB, Wood PC, et al. Does melatonin improve sleep in older people? A randomised crossover trial. Age Ageing 2003;32(2):164–70.

[45] Singer C, Tractenberg RE, Kaye J, et al. A multicenter, placebo-controlled trial of melatonin for sleep disturbance in Alzheimer's disease. Sleep 2003;26(7):893–901.

[46] Zhdanova IV, Wurtman RJ, Regan MM, et al. Melatonin treatment for age-related insomnia. J Clin Endocrinol Metab 2001;86(10):4727–30.

[47] Monti JM, Alvarino D, Cardinali D, et al. Polysomnographic study of the effect of melatonin on sleep in elderly patients with chronic primary insomnia. Arch Gerontol Geriatr 1999;28:85–98.

[48] Hughes RJ, Sack RL, Lewy AJ. The role of melatonin and circadian phase in age-related sleep-maintenance insomnia: assessment in a clinical trial of melatonin replacement. Sleep 1998;21(1):52–68.

[49] Dawson D, Rogers NL, van den Heuvel CJ, et al. Effect of sustained nocturnal transbuccal melatonin administration on sleep and temperature in elderly insomniacs. J Biol Rhythms 1998;13(6):532–8.

[50] Buscemi N, Vandermeer B, Pandya R, et al. Melatonin for Treatment of Sleep Disorders, Evidence Report/Technology Assessment No. 108. Rockville, MD: agency for Healthcare Research and Quality. Prepared by the University of Alberta Evidence-based Practice Center, under Contract No. 290-02-0023; November 2004. AHRQ Publication No. 05-E002-2.

[51] Haimov I, Lavie P, Laudon M, et al. Melatonin replacement therapy of elderly insomniacs. Sleep 1995;18(7):598–603.

[52] Leger D, Laudon M, Zisapel N. Nocturnal 6-sulfatoxymelatonin excretion in insomnia and its relation to the response to melatonin replacement therapy. Am J Med 2004; 116(2):91–5.

[53] Siegrist C, Benedetti C, Orlando A, et al. Lack of changes in serum prolactin, FSH, TSH, and estradiol after melatonin treatment in doses that improve sleep and reduce benzodiazepine consumption in sleep-disturbed, middle-aged, and elderly patients. J Pineal Res 2001; 30(1):34–42.

[54] Seabra ML, Bignotto M, Pinto LR Jr, et al. Randomized, double-blind clinical trial, controlled with placebo, of the toxicology of chronic melatonin treatment. J Pineal Res 2000; 29(4):193–200.

[55] Buscemi N, Vandermeer B, Hooton N, et al. The efficacy and safety of exogenous melatonin for primary sleep disorders. A meta-analysis. J Gen Intern Med 2005;20(12):1151–8.

[56] Mendelson WB. A critical evaluation of the hypnotic efficacy of melatonin. Sleep 1997; 20(10):916–9.

[57] Rogers NL, Phan O, Kennaway DJ, et al. Effect of daytime oral melatonin administration on neurobehavioral performance in humans. J Pineal Res 1998;25(1):47–53.

[58] Okawa M, Uchiyama M, Ozaki S, et al. Melatonin treatment for circadian rhythm sleep disorders. Psychiatry Clin Neurosci 1998;52(2):259–60.

[59] Middleton BA, Stone BM, Arendt J. Melatonin and fragmented sleep patterns. Lancet 1996;348(9026):551–2.

[60] Dawson D, van den Heuvel CJ. Integrating the actions of melatonin on human physiology. Ann Med 1998;30(1):95–102.

[61] Lusardi P, Piazza E, Fogari R. Cardiovascular effects of melatonin in hypertensive patients well controlled by nifedipine: a 24-hour study. Br J Clin Pharmacol 2000;49(5):423–7.

[62] Sewerynek E. Melatonin and the cardiovascular system. Neuroendocrinol Lett 2002; 23(Suppl 1):79–83.

[63] Maestroni GJ. The immunotherapeutic potential of melatonin. Expert Opin Investig Drugs 2001;10(3):467–76.

[64] Hansson I, Holmdahl R, Mattsson R. Constant darkness enhances autoimmunity to type II collagen and exaggerates development of collagen-induced arthritis in DBA/1 mice. J Neuroimmunol 1990;27(1):79–84.

[65] Maestroni GJ, Sulli A, Pizzorni C, et al. Melatonin in rheumatoid arthritis: synovial macrophages show melatonin receptors. Ann N Y Acad Sci 2002;966:271–5.

[66] Conti A, Maestroni GJ. Melatonin rhythms in mice: role in autoimmune and lymphoproliferative diseases. Ann N Y Acad Sci 1998;840:395–410.

[67] Bilici D, Akpinar E, Kiziltunc A. Protective effect of melatonin in carrageenan-induced acute local inflammation. Pharmacol Res 2002;46(2):133–9.

[68] Hong YG, Riegler JL. Is melatonin associated with the development of autoimmune hepatitis? J Clin Gastroenterol 1997;25(1):376–8.

[69] Medical Letter. Melatonin. Med Lett Drugs Ther 1995;37(962):111–2.

[70] Leibenluft E, Feldman-Naim S, Turner EH, et al. Effects of exogenous melatonin administration and withdrawal in five patients with rapid-cycling bipolar disorder. J Clin Psychiatry 1997;58(9):383–8.

[71] Maksoud A, Moore CA, Harshkowitz M. The effect of melatonin administration on patients with sleep apnea. Sleep Research 1997;26:114.

[72] Olde Rikkert MG, Rigaud AS. Melatonin in elderly patients with insomnia. A systematic review. Z Gerontol Geriatr 2001;34(6):491–7.

[73] Bellipanni G, Bianchi P, Pierpaoli W, et al. Effects of melatonin in perimenopausal and menopausal women: a randomized and placebo controlled study. Exp Gerontol 2001; 36(2):297–310.

[74] Attele AS, Xie JT, Yuan CS. Treatment of insomnia: an alternative approach. Altern Med Rev 2000;5(3):249–59.

[75] Pawlikowski M, Kolomecka M, Wojtczak A, et al. Effects of six months melatonin treatment on sleep quality and serum concentrations of estradiol, cortisol, dehydroepiandrosterone sulfate, and somatomedin C in elderly women. Neuroendocrinol Lett 2002;23(Suppl 1): 17–9.

[76] National Academies–Committee on the Framework for Evaluating the Safety of Dietary Supplements. Prototype Monograph on Melatonin. Dietary supplements: a framework for evaluation safety. Washington, D.C.: The National Academies Press; 2004. p. D1–71.

[77] Houghton PJ. The scientific basis for the reputed activity of Valerian. J Pharm Pharmacol 1999;51(5):505–12.

[78] Santos MS, Ferreira F, Cunha AP, et al. Synaptosomal GABA release as influenced by valerian root extract—involvement of the GABA carrier. Arch Int Pharmacodyn Ther 1994;327(2):220–31.

[79] Muller CE, Schumacher B, Brattstrom A, et al. Interactions of valerian extracts and a fixed valerian-hop extract combination with adenosine receptors. Life Sci 2002;71(16): 1939–49.

[80] Dietz BM, Mahady GB, Pauli GF, et al. Valerian extract and valerenic acid are partial agonists of the 5-HT5a receptor in vitro. Brain Res Mol Brain Res 2005;138(2):191–7.

[81] ConsumerLab.com. Valerian: product review. Available at: www.consumerlab.com. Accessed May 20, 2007.

[82] Balderer G, Borbely AA. Effect of valerian on human sleep. Psychopharmacology 1985; 87(4):406–9.

[83] Leathwood PD, Chauffard F. Aqueous extract of valerian reduces latency to fall asleep in man. Planta Med 1985;51(2):144–8.

[84] Donath F, Quispe S, Diefenbach K, et al. Critical evaluation of the effect of valerian extract on sleep structure and sleep quality. Pharmacopsychiatry 2000;33(2):47–53.

[85] Leathwood PD, Chauffard F, Heck E, et al. Aqueous extract of valerian root (Valeriana officinalis L.) improves sleep quality in man. Pharmacol Biochem Behav 1982;17(1):65–71.

[86] Poyares DR, Guilleminault C, Ohayon MM, et al. Can valerian improve the sleep of insomniacs after benzodiazepine withdrawal? Prog Neuropsychopharmacol Biol Psychiatry 2002; 26(3):539–45.

[87] Ziegler G, Ploch M, Miettinen-Baumann A, et al. Efficacy and tolerability of valerian extract LI 156 compared with oxazepam in the treatment of non-organic insomnia—a randomized, double-blind, comparative clinical study. Eur J Med Res 2002;7(11):480–6.

[88] Schulz H, Stolz C, Muller J. The effect of valerian extract on sleep polygraphy in poor sleepers: a pilot study. Pharmacopsychiatry 1994;27(4):147–51.

[89] Diaper A, Hindmarch I. A double-blind, placebo-controlled investigation of the effects of two doses of a valerian preparation on the sleep, cognitive and psychomotor function of sleep-disturbed older adults. Phytother Res 2004;18(10):831–6.

[90] PDR for Herbal Remedies. Montvale (NJ): Medical Economics; 1998.

[91] Morin CM, Koetter U, Bastien C, et al. Valerian-hops combination and diphenhydramine for treating insomnia: a randomized placebo-controlled clinical trial. Sleep 2005;28(11): 1465–71.

[92] Block KI, Gyllenhaal C, Mead MN. Safety and efficacy of herbal sedatives in cancer care. Integr Cancer Ther 2004;3(2):128–48.

[93] Taibi DM, Bourguignon C, Taylor AG. Valerian use for sleep disturbances related to rheumatoid arthritis. Holist Nurs Pract 2004;18(3):120–6.

[94] Richards K, Nagel C, Markie M, et al. Use of complementary and alternative therapies to promote sleep in critically ill patients. Crit Care Nurs Clin North Am 2003;15(3):329–40.

[95] Plushner SL. Valerian: valeriana officinalis. Am J Health Syst Pharm 2000;57(4):328, 333, 335.

[96] Kuhlmann J, Berger W, Podzuweit H, et al. The influence of valerian treatment on "reaction time, alertness and concentration" in volunteers. Pharmacopsychiatry 1999; 32(6):235–41.

[97] Garges HP, Varia I, Doraiswamy PM. Cardiac complications and delirium associated with valerian root withdrawal [letter]. JAMA 1998;280(18):1566–7.

[98] Soden K, Vincent K, Craske S, et al. A randomized controlled trial of aromatherapy massage in a hospice setting. Palliat Med 2004;18(2):87–92.

[99] Hanley J, Stirling P, Brown C. Randomised controlled trial of therapeutic massage in the management of stress. Br J Gen Pract 2003;53(486):20–5.

[100] McDowell JA, Mion LC, Lydon TJ, et al. A nonpharmacologic sleep protocol for hospitalized older patients. J Am Geriatr Soc 1998;46(6):700–5.

[101] Richards KC. Effect of a back massage and relaxation intervention on sleep in critically ill patients. Am J Crit Care 1998;7(4):288–99.

[102] Field T, Diego M, Cullen C, et al. Fibromyalgia Pain and substance p decrease and sleep improves after massage therapy. J Clin Rheumatol 2002;8(2):72–6.

[103] Sarac AJ, Gur A. Complementary and alternative medical therapies in fibromyalgia. Curr Pharm Des 2006;12(1):47–57.

[104] Chen ML, Lin LC, Wu SC, et al. The effectiveness of acupressure in improving the quality of sleep of institutionalized residents. J Gerontol A Biol Sci Med Sci 1999;54(8):M389–94.

[105] Tsay SL, Chen ML. Acupressure and quality of sleep in patients with end-stage renal disease—a randomized controlled trial. Int J Nurs Stud 2003;40(1):1–7.

[106] Tsay SL, Cho YC, Chen ML. Acupressure and Transcutaneous Electrical Acupoint Stimulation in improving fatigue, sleep quality and depression in hemodialysis patients. Am J Chin Med 2004;32(3):407–16.

[107] Yang MH, Wu SC, Lin JG, et al. The efficacy of acupressure for decreasing agitated behaviour in dementia: a pilot study. J Clin Nurs 2007;16(2):308–15.

[108] Suen LK, Wong TK, Leung AW, et al. The long-term effects of auricular therapy using magnetic pearls on elderly with insomnia. Complement Ther Med 2003;11(2):85–92.

[109] Suen LK, Wong TK, Leung AW. Effectiveness of auricular therapy on sleep promotion in the elderly. Am J Chin Med 2002;30(4):429–49.

[110] Spence DW, Kayumov L, Chen A, et al. Acupuncture increases nocturnal melatonin secretion and reduces insomnia and anxiety: a preliminary report. J Neuropsychiatry Clin Neurosci 2004;16(1):19–28.

[111] Montakab H. [Acupuncture and insomnia]. Forsch Komplementarmed 1999;6(Suppl 1): 29–31.

[112] Kim YS, Lee SH, Jung WS, et al. Intradermal acupuncture on shen-men and nei-kuan acupoints in patients with insomnia after stroke. Am J Chin Med 2004;32(5):771–8.

[113] Huang MI, Nir Y, Chen B, et al. A randomized controlled pilot study of acupuncture for postmenopausal hot flashes: effect on nocturnal hot flashes and sleep quality. Fertil Steril 2006;86(3):700–10.

[114] Carpenter JS, Neal JG. Other complementary and alternative medicine modalities: acupuncture, magnets, reflexology, and homeopathy. Am J Med 2005;118(Suppl 12B): 109–17.

[115] Rooks DS. Fibromyalgia treatment update. Curr Opin Rheumatol 2007;19(2):111–7.

[116] Holdcraft LC, Assefi N, Buchwald D. Complementary and alternative medicine in fibromyalgia and related syndromes. Best Pract Res Clin Rheumatol 2003;17(4):667–83.

[117] Freire AO, Sugai GC, Chrispin FS, et al. Treatment of moderate obstructive sleep apnea syndrome with acupuncture: a randomised, placebo-controlled pilot trial. Sleep Med 2007;8(1):43–50.

[118] Wang XH, Yuan YD, Wang BF. [Clinical observation on effect of auricular acupoint pressing in treating sleep apnea syndrome]. Zhongguo Zhong Xi Yi Jie He Za Zhi 2003; 23(10):747–9.

[119] Mason LI, Alexander CN, Travis FT, et al. Electrophysiological correlates of higher states of consciousness during sleep in long-term practitioners of the Transcendental Meditation program. Sleep 1997;20(2):102–10.

[120] Smith JE, Richardson J, Hoffman C, et al. Mindfulness-Based Stress Reduction as supportive therapy in cancer care: systematic review. J Adv Nurs 2005;52(3):315–27.

[121] Carlson LE, Garland SN. Impact of mindfulness-based stress reduction (MBSR) on sleep, mood, stress and fatigue symptoms in cancer outpatients. Int J Behav Med 2005;12(4): 278–85.

[122] Manjunath NK, Telles S. Influence of Yoga and Ayurveda on self-rated sleep in a geriatric population. Indian J Med Res 2005;121(5):683–90.

[123] Cohen L, Warneke C, Fouladi RT, et al. Psychological adjustment and sleep quality in a randomized trial of the effects of a Tibetan yoga intervention in patients with lymphoma. Cancer 2004;100(10):2253–60.

[124] Bower JE, Woolery A, Sternlieb B, et al. Yoga for cancer patients and survivors. Cancer Control 2005;12(3):165–71.

[125] Li F, Fisher KJ, Harmer P, et al. Tai Chi and self-rated quality of sleep and daytime sleepiness in older adults: a randomized controlled trial. J Am Geriatr Soc 2004;52(6): 892–900.

ELSEVIER
SAUNDERS

CLINICS IN
GERIATRIC
MEDICINE

Clin Geriatr Med 24 (2008) 139–149

Light Therapy for Insomnia in Older Adults

Julie K. Gammack, MD[a,b,*]

[a]Division of Geriatric Medicine, Saint Louis University Health Sciences Center,
1402 S. Grand Boulevard, M238, St. Louis, MO 63104, USA
[b]Geriatric Research Education and Clinical Center (GRECC), Jefferson Barracks Veteran's
Affairs Medical Center, 1 Jefferson Barracks Drive, St. Louis, MO 63125-4199, USA

Insomnia is the subjective report of inadequate or nonrestorative sleep, despite adequate opportunity to get proper rest. Insomnia may be a primary disorder, or may be secondary to physical, medical, or psychosocial factors. Older adults are at risk for primary sleep disorders, such as restless legs syndrome and sleep apnea, but are also at risk for secondary sleep disorders caused by the accumulation of diseases and illnesses that impair proper sleep.

Treatment for insomnia frequently relies on pharmacotherapy interventions. Nonpharmacotherapy approaches, such as improved sleep hygiene, cognitive-behavioral therapy, and management of contributing comorbidities, are underutilized and can be quite effective. The contribution of dark-light cycles in regulating sleep patterns is infrequently considered as an environmental contributor to poor sleep. Adequate bright light exposure is necessary for sleep regulation; it is both a nonpharmacologic and a pharmacologic factor, via melatonin regulation, in maintaining the natural circadian rhythm.

Older adults are less likely than younger adults to receive prolonged, high intensity, daily bright light exposure. Institutionalized, frail, and chronically ill elders are less likely to have bright light exposure than healthy elders. Chronic illnesses, such as dementia and depression, are frequent in this elderly population and contribute to both poor sleep and limited bright light exposure.

The use of bright light therapy (BLT) to treat sleep disorders in demented and depressed elders may reduce unwanted behavioral and cognitive

* Division of Geriatric Medicine, Saint Louis University Health Sciences Center, 1402 S. Grand Boulevard, M238, St. Louis, MO 63104.

E-mail address: gammackj@slu.edu

0749-0690/08/$ - see front matter © 2008 Elsevier Inc. All rights reserved.
doi:10.1016/j.cger.2007.08.013   *geriatric.theclinics.com*

symptoms. Conversely, treating demented and depressed individuals with bright light may reduce the effects of these conditions on the sleep-wake cycle. This article reviews the current evidence for BLT in older adults, for insomnia and cognitive conditions that adversely affect sleep.

Principles of light therapy

The circadian rhythm

It is well established that a person's circadian rhythm is strongly influenced by exposure to light. The circadian rhythm is regulated by the suprachiasmatic nuclei (SCN) in the hypothalamus. This center regulates rhythms that promote sleeping and wakening. The natural length of the circadian clock is just over 24 hours. When light enters the retina, it activates photoreceptor neurons leading to the SCN. The SCN responds to these impulses by stimulating the production of melatonin by the pineal gland. Research suggests that melatonin is a major regulator of the circadian rhythm and core body temperature. Melatonin secretion and core body temperature are inversely related. In normal adults, the body temperature minimum occurs 1 to 2 hours before awakening, generally between 4 AM and 5 AM. This corresponds to the maximal concentration of circulating melatonin levels [1]. Core body temperature and melatonin are the two primary and measurable markers of the circadian cycle.

Melatonin

Melatonin is a neuroendocrine hormone released by the pineal gland via diffusion into the bloodstream. The synthesis and release of melatonin is stimulated by darkness and inhibited by light in a dose-dependent fashion. Inhibition threshold is between 200 lux and 400 lux (ambient indoor fluorescent light), and maximal inhibition occurs at 600 lux after 60 minutes [2]. Melatonin levels rise shortly after dark and peak between 2 AM and 4 AM With aging, there is evidence that maximal melatonin levels decrease at night and that the rise in melatonin occurs 60 to 90 minutes earlier than in younger adults [3]. There is also evidence that low melatonin levels may be present in adults with more severe depressive symptoms [4].

Altering the circadian rhythm

It is possible to adjust the natural circadian rhythm by light exposure, shifting sleep schedules, and pharmacotherapy (such as melatonin). Scheduled light exposure at consistent intervals greater than or less than 24 hours results in a phase-shift of melatonin production and of the core body temperature rhythm. This in turn alters the endogenous circadian rhythm of sleep and wakefulness.

The timing of treatment is important when sleep-phase cycle disturbances, jet lag, or shift work require a resetting of the natural circadian
rhythm. Light exposure may be provided at different times of the day, based
on the sleep disorder being treated. There is some research to suggest that
scheduling light or dark periods promotes adaptation to shift work [5,6].
In older adults, Leproult and colleagues [7] induced a phase-advancement
in core body temperature of nearly 2 hours, with the administration of
a melatonin agonist. Although neurohormonal patterns were also altered,
there was no effect on any sleep parameter in this study.

Bright light therapy

Most research on BLT has focused on the sleep-wake disturbances of jet
lag and shift work adaptation and on depression (both seasonal affective
disorder and nonseasonal depression). In the elderly population, BLT has
also been studied in managing behavioral disturbances and other nocturnal
sleep disruptions in demented and institutionalized individuals.

There is no consensus on the optimum treatment protocol for BLT. Most
studies administer a light intensity of 2000 lux to 10,000 lux, for 30 to 120
minutes daily, over 7 to 28 days. Virtually all studies administer BLT via
an artificial light box, as opposed to natural light exposure. The administration time for BLT is usually morning (7 AM–9 AM) or evening (7 PM–9 PM);
however, some studies have provided treatment during the mid-day. There is
no consensus on the best time of day for administering BLT for depression
or dementia-related symptoms. Potential side effects of BLT include headache, nausea, dry skin, and eye symptoms including dryness, sensitivity,
and vascular injection of eye tissues. In healthy older adults, bright light
therapy may result in irritability, anxiousness, and agitation [8].

In clinical studies, sleep parameters are usually measured using a variety
of tools, including sleep surveys, sleep diaries, direct observation, polysomnography, and actigraphy. Actigraphy is the measurement of gross motor
activity using an accelerometer, usually on the wrist. Motor activity and
the absence of motor activity are surrogate markers for the state of wakefulness or sleep, respectively.

The American Academy of Sleep Medicine (AASM) has published practice
parameters for the use of BLT in the treatment of sleep disorders (Table 1).
These recommendations are based on review of the medical literature and
are graded based on the strength of the evidence. A "Standard" recommendation is given to generally accepted care with a high degree of clinical certainty
and high quality evidence (randomized trials). A "Guideline" recommendation reflects a moderate degree of clinical certainty based on cohort, randomized, and nonrandomized trials. An "Option" recommendation reflects
uncertain clinical utility based on inconclusive or conflicting evidence. The
conditions reviewed by the AASM include delayed and advanced sleep phase
syndrome, non-24-hour sleep-wake syndrome, irregular sleep-wake disorder,

Table 1
American Academy of Sleep Medicine practice parameters for light therapy

Recommendation	Strength of evidence
A prescribing physician should be aware of dosage recommendations, potential side effects, and recommended light intensity limits if light therapy is to be used.	Standard
Light therapy appears to be a generally safe treatment option for some circadian rhythm disorders when used within reported guidelines for light intensity and time limits.	Guideline
Light therapy appears to have potential utility based on current study data in the treatment of delayed sleep phase syndrome (DSPS).	Guideline
The minimum or optimal duration of light therapy for DSPS is unknown.	Option
Light therapy appears to have potential utility based on current study data in the treatment of advanced sleep phase syndrome (ASPS).	Guideline
The minimum or optimal duration of light therapy for ASPS is unknown.	Option
Light therapy may be of benefit in treating some blind patients with non-24-hour sleep-wake syndrome.	Option
The minimum duration of light therapy for non-24-hour sleep-wake syndrome is unknown.	Option
While the evidence is minimal and sometimes conflicting, bright light exposure at destination to enhance circadian re-entrainment would appear safe and potentially beneficial for travelers across multiple time zones.	Option
Bright light before the core body temperature minimum may be helpful in shifting workers from a day to evening to night rotation work schedule.	Opinion
Bright light after the core body temperature minimum may be helpful in shifting workers from a night to evening to day schedule.	Option
Adequate studies are not available to provide specific recommendations on light therapy to treat other causes of insomnia in healthy elderly.	
No specific recommendation is made about the clinical use of light therapy in dementia patients.	

shift work, jet lag, secondary insomnia from depression, and insomnia in both healthy and demented elders [9].

Light therapy for insomnia

Healthy elders

There is some limited evidence that BLT is helpful in improving sleep quality in healthy older adults without insomnia symptoms [10–12]. In one study, eight healthy women (mean age 67 years) received 1 hour of morning light therapy each day for 1 week, followed by a crossover to nonlight therapy for 1 week. Sleep parameters were recorded using self-report and wrist actigraphy. By treatment day two, self-reported motivation, happiness, alertness, mood, refreshment, and appetite were significantly improved ($P < .05$). By day four, sleep maintenance, anxiety, and integrated sleep feeling was improved ($P < .05$) [10].

The data on BLT efficacy in healthy older adults with insomnia is equally limited. Suhner and colleagues [13] studied 15 older adults with chronic insomnia. These participants received daily evening BLT for up to 14 days, followed by twice-weekly maintenance therapy for 2 months. Although a phase delay in the minimum core body temperature of 94 minutes was noted, sleep quality was not improved during the maintenance phase in control or treatment groups.

In another study, 31 subjects age 55 years or older, who suffered from mild early morning awakening, were randomized to bright light, dim light, or placebo treatment. Light exposure took place daily in the evening in the patients' homes, 30 to 60 minutes before bedtime for 3 weeks. Sleep parameters were recorded using a sleep diary and wrist actigraphy. Of the eight self-reported sleep outcomes and six actigraphic sleep variables assessed, only "time spent in bed after final morning awakening" significantly improved at the end of the study compared with baseline in the treatment group [14].

A meta-analyses was performed to evaluate the efficacy of BLT in improving sleep quality among adults aged 60 and above. This Cochrane Collaboration Report evaluated the effect of sleep quality in nondemented individuals [15]. The investigators found no trials on which to base conclusions for the effectiveness of this treatment, and thus concluded that "When the possible side-effects of standard treatment (hypnotics) are considered, there is a reasonable argument to be made for clinical use of non-pharmacological treatments. In view of the promising results of bright light therapy in other populations with problems of sleep timing, further research into their effectiveness with older adults would seem justifiable."

Demented elders

Older adults with dementia are at higher risk of developing sleep disturbances than nondemented individuals. Distinguishing between sleep-related and dementia-related behavioral disturbances can be difficult, so a nonpharmacologic intervention, such as BLT, that can improve both conditions would be quite beneficial. A meta-analyses was performed to evaluate the efficacy of BLT in the categories of managing sleep, behavior, mood, and cognitive disturbances associated with dementia [16]. A review of the literature revealed three studies of sufficient quality for further analysis. These studies were of significant heterogeneity, which prevented pooling of data and the study design prevented further subgroup analysis for the above categories. The investigators thus concluded that there was insufficient conclusive evidence on of the benefit of light therapy [16].

Many older adults with dementia reside at home with the assistance of family, caregivers, or social service providers. Reducing sleep disturbance is important for the health and quality of life for both caregivers and care-receivers. Reducing sleep disturbances can reduce the likelihood of institutionalization [17].

In a randomized controlled trial, McCurry and colleagues [18] studied primary sleep outcomes in 36 community-dwelling patients with Alzheimer's disease, using sleep surveys and wrist actigraphy. Patient-caregiver pairs received dementia education and then were randomized to either daily exercise plus 60 minutes of BLT or to usual care (control) for 2 months. At 2 months, the treatment group showed significantly greater ($P < .05$) reductions in number of nighttime awakenings, total time awake at night, and depression, compared with control subjects. At the 6-month follow-up, sleep parameter benefits were maintained, and additional significant improvement in duration of night awakenings was seen. After controlling for severity of cognitive impairment, the treatment group had less daytime sleepiness than controls throughout the study.

The institutional setting

Many nursing home residents have difficulty sleeping at night. Sleep disturbance in this population is characterized by frequent nocturnal awakenings, sleep latency of greater than 30 minutes, and prolonged time spent in bed. Poor sleep can lead to confusion, poor control of medical illnesses, and impaired rehabilitation. These adults face many barriers to restful and sufficient sleep. In addition to multiple comorbid conditions that affect sleep, institutionalized elders are less likely than community dwellers to have a sufficient bright light exposure for regulation of the circadian rhythm. In one study of 66 institutionalized adults, the average light exposure intensity was 54 lux, and the median exposure time to light over 1000 lux was only 10.5 minutes each day [19]. As mentioned above, sufficient intensity and duration of light exposure is necessary to properly regulate melatonin secretion and the circadian rhythm.

Several studies have been performed to evaluate the use of bright light therapy on the sleep patterns of demented, institutionalized elders. Fetveit and Bjorvatn [20] administered 2 hours of daily morning bright light for 2 weeks in 11 demented adults with sleep-wake disturbance. Nursing reports and wrist actigraphy were used to quantify sleep parameters for up to 16 weeks posttreatment. Daytime nap duration was significantly reduced by 30 minutes during the treatment period ($P = .004$), but this effect was not sustained after cessation of light therapy. Other research suggests that the effects of BLT on sleep may be sustained from 4 to 8 weeks after treatment cessation [21]. In a similarly designed study by the same investigtors, participants receiving light therapy had greater sleep efficiency (85% versus 73%), decreased sleep latency (17 minutes versus 1 hour 17 minutes), wake time after sleep onset (1 hour, 23 minutes versus 1 hour, 49 minutes), decreased early morning awakenings (1 minute versus 16 minutes), decreased time in bed (11 hours, 56 minutes versus 12 hours, 32 minutes), decreased total wake time (1 hour, 40 minutes versus 3 hours, 24 minutes), and increased total sleep time (10 hours, 12 minutes versus 9 hours, 10 minutes) during treatment when compared with pre-treatment parameters (all $P < .05$) [22].

In a larger randomized controlled study by Ancoli-Israel and colleagues [23], 77 nursing home residents with dementia (mean age 86 years) received 2 hours of either morning bright light, evening bright light, evening dim light, or placebo for 18 days. Sleep parameters were measured with wrist actigraphy. In this study, nighttime sleep and daytime alertness were unchanged in the treatment groups; however, morning light was found to delay the peak circadian rhythm activity and increase mean activity level, compared with baseline ($P < .05$).

The same authors studied 92 demented, nursing home elders who received 120 minutes of morning bright light, morning dim light, evening bright light, or placebo over 10 days. Sleep parameters were measured with wrist actigraphy and direct observation. In this study, maximal sleep duration increased from 65 minutes to 88 minutes in the morning bright light group, and from 71 minutes to 95 minutes in the evening bright light group when compared with baseline. ($P \leq .05$) [24]. Expanding on this intervention, the same subjects were evaluated for agitated behaviors before, during, and after treatment. Morning bright light delayed the onset of agitated behaviors by 1.5 hours.

Multidimensional therapy

Light therapy may be used in combination with other nonpharmacologic methods to improve sleep quality. This approach requires a coordinated effort between physicians, nurses, therapists, and activity staff. This type of program usually includes an exposure to bright light during the morning or evening, and a combination of other strategies such as daytime activities to maintain wakefulness, a structured sleep hygiene program, noise reduction, and a consistent bedtime care routine.

Two recent trials have looked at the use of light therapy as a component of a multidimensional method of improving sleep quality in the nursing home setting. Alessi and colleagues [25] randomized 118 demented elderly nursing home residents to a structured behavioral and activity program, including 30 minutes of morning bright light daily for 5 days. Sleep and behaviors were measured with direct observations and wrist actigraphy. The treatment group was significantly less likely to be asleep during the day (32% versus 21% of observations) at completion compared with baseline.

In another study, 173 demented nursing home residents were provided increased daytime physical activity, evening bright light therapy, noise reduction, and bedtime and nighttime routines. Sleep parameters were measured with wrist actigraphy, polysomnography, and direct observations. When treated, participants were more likely to be awake during the day when compared with baseline [26]. Unfortunately, no other measures of daytime or nighttime sleep activity were significantly changed with this intervention.

Light therapy for behavioral symptoms

Agitated behaviors are common in demented residents of chronic care facilities. Agitation may be linked to the sleep-wake cycle, thus evaluating the effect of bright light on sleep symptoms in demented elders may also provide information on behavioral disturbances. The evidence for improvement in agitation in demented elders with the use of BLT is mixed.

In one randomized controlled crossover study, 15 institutionalized elders with dementia and agitated behaviors received 1 hour of BLT daily versus control for 4 weeks. Participants were then crossed over to the other treatment arm. Those receiving light therapy had a significant improvement from baseline in sleep duration, with an average of 8.1 hours per night versus 6.4 hours per night ($P < .05$). The control group did not improve. There were no improvements in agitated behaviors during the study [27].

In another study, 10 demented elders with both sleep disturbance and behavioral symptoms were given 45 minutes of bright light therapy each morning for 4 weeks. Sleep and behavioral symptoms were recorded using wrist actigraphy and direct observation, respectively. In this study, no improvement in sleep parameters was seen but behavioral symptoms improved on two clinical rating scales, both during and after treatment [28].

Mishima and colleagues [29] evaluated 14 hospitalized elders with dementia showing sleep and behavior disorders, and 10 controls (average age 75 years). Participants were observed for behavioral disturbances before, during, and after a 4-week, daily, morning BLT protocol. The average behavioral disturbance score decreased significantly in the BLT group during treatment compared with baseline. Several sleep parameters were significantly improved in the treated group during BLT (total sleep time, nocturnal sleep time, daytime sleep time) compared with baseline, but these effects were not sustained after completion of the BLT protocol.

The largest study of BLT for behavioral management of demented elders included 92 institutionalized individuals who were randomized to morning bright or dim light, evening bright light, or placebo. Agitation was rated every 15 minutes and pre- and posttreatment. Those receiving bright light had a 1.5-hour delay in onset of agitated behavior, but no difference was found on agitation severity ratings [30].

Light therapy for depression

The benefits of BLT therapy extend beyond sleep cycle improvement. It is well known that the mood symptoms of depression, specifically seasonal affective disorder, can be improved with BLT [31–33]. Because sleep disturbance is a common symptom of, and one of the Diagnostic and Statistical Manual of Mental Disorders, fourth edition, diagnostic criteria for, major depressive disorder, the use of BLT in depressed individuals may have benefit on both mood symptoms and on sleep.

BLT has been studied specifically in nonseasonal depression but has demonstrated less robust benefit than for seasonal depression. A 2004 Cochrane Database analysis of light therapy for nonseasonal depression reported no consensus on its efficacy. Twenty studies were identified, most of which used BLT in conjunction with pharmacotherapy. In general, the quality of evidence was poor. Although the results of BLT were better than control treatment, they did not reach statistical significance. Only when those studies of highest research quality were pooled were the results of BLT significantly better than control (standardized mean difference: -0.90; 95% confidence interval or CI, -1.50 to -0.31) [34].

A meta-analysis of light therapy in the treatment of mood disorders published the following year by Golden and colleagues [35], reported predominantly positive benefits of BLT. For all depressive types, BLT significantly reduced depression symptom severity with an effect size of 0.84 (95% CI, 0.60–1.08). BLT also significantly reduced depressive symptoms for nonseasonal depression (0.53; 95% CI, 0.18–0.89) and for seasonal depression (0.73; 95% CI, 0.37–1.08). BLT was not found to significantly reduce depressive symptoms when used in conjunction with pharmacotherapy for depression management.

BLT may be beneficial in the treatment of depression in hospitalized elders. In one study, 60 hospitalized individuals (average age 75 years) were randomized to 5 days of 5000 lux morning, artificial light versus control. Geriatric depression scale (GDS) scores were similar at baseline between groups. With treatment, GDS scores dropped significantly ($P < .001$) by 5 points to 13.1 (standard deviation plus or minus 3.5) but did not change in control groups [36].

Depressive symptoms may also improve in institutionalized older adults treated with BLT. In a placebo-controlled study, 14 participants (mean age 84 years) received 5 days of bright light, dim light, or no light therapy. GDS scores decreased significantly during the BLT (pretest GDS equals 15 versus posttest GDS equals 11, $P < .01$) but did not change during the dim- or no-light period. After BLT, 50% of the participants no longer scored in the depressed range [37].

Summary

Exposure to bright light suppresses the production of melatonin and contributes to the regulation of the circadian rhythm. Because of environmental and medical conditions, older adults are less likely than younger adults to receive the prolonged, high intensity, daily, bright light needed to promote a satisfactory sleep-wake cycle. The best available evidence for BLT is in the management of seasonal affective disorder, which is relatively infrequent in the elderly population. For older adults with chronic insomnia, dementia, and nonseasonal depression, there is no consensus on the optimum treatment protocol for BLT. Much of the research on BLT in these conditions is of limited quality and of mixed results. In addition to sleep improvement, BLT may reduce unwanted behavioral and cognitive symptoms. Conversely, treating demented and depressed individuals with bright light may reduce the effects of these conditions on the sleep-wake cycle.

References

[1] Cagnacci A, Elliott JA, Yen SS. Melatonin: a major regulator of the circadian rhythm of core temperature in humans. J Clin Endocrinol Metab 1992;75(2):447–52.
[2] McIntyre IM, Norman TR, Burrows GD, et al. Quantal melatonin suppression by exposure to low intensity light in man. Life Sci 1989;45(4):327–32.
[3] van Coevorden A, Mockel J, Laurent E, et al. Neuroendocrine rhythms and sleep in aging men. Am J Physiol 1991;260(4 Pt 1):E651–61.
[4] Brown RP, Kocsis JH, Caroff S, et al. Depressed mood and reality disturbance correlate with decreased nocturnal melatonin in depressed patients. Acta Psychiatr Scand 1987;76(3): 272–5.
[5] Santhi N, Duffy JF, Horowitz TS, et al. Scheduling of sleep/darkness affects the circadian phase of night shift workers. Neurosci Lett 2005;384(3):316–20.
[6] Yoon IY, Song BG. Role of morning melatonin administration and attenuation of sunlight exposure in improving adaptation of night-shift workers. Chronobiol Int 2002;19(5):903–13.
[7] Leproult R, Van Onderbergen A, L'hermite-Balériaux M, et al. Phase-shifts of 24-h rhythms of hormonal release and body temperature following early evening administration of the melatonin agonist agomelatine in healthy older men. Clin Endocrinol (Oxf) 2005;63(3):298–304.
[8] Genhart MJ, Kelly KA, Coursey RD, et al. Effects of bright light on mood in normal elderly women. Psychiatry Res 1993;47(1):87–97.
[9] Chesson AL, Littner M, Davila D, et al. Practice parameters for the use of light therapy in the treatment of sleep disorders. Sleep 1999;22(5):641–60.
[10] Kohsaka M, Fukuda N, Honma H, et al. Effects of moderately bright light on subjective evaluations in healthy elderly women. Psychiatry Clin Neurosci 1999;53(2):239–41.
[11] Kobayashi R, Kohsaka M, Fukuda N, et al. Effects of morning bright light on sleep in healthy elderly women. Psychiatry Clin Neurosci 1999;53(2):237–8.
[12] Kohsaka M, Fukuda N, Kobayashi R, et al. Effect of short duration morning bright light in elderly men: sleep structure. Psychiatry Clin Neurosci 2000;54(3):367–8.
[13] Suhner AG, Murphy PJ, Campbell SS. Failure of timed bright light exposure to alleviate age-related sleep maintenance insomnia. J Am Geriatr Soc 2002;50(4):617–23.
[14] Pallesen S, Nordhus IH, Skelton SH, et al. Bright light treatment has limited effect in subjects over 55 years with mild early morning awakening. Percept Mot Skills 2005;101(3):759–70.
[15] Montgomery P, Dennis J. Bright light therapy for sleep problems in adults aged 60+. [Systematic Review] Cochrane Developmental, Psychosocial and Learning Problems Group Cochrane Database of Systematic Reviews 2007;3:CD003403.
[16] Forbes D, Morgan DG, Bangma J, et al. Light therapy for managing sleep, behaviour, and mood disturbances in dementia. Cochrane Dementia and Cognitive Improvement Group Cochrane Database of Systematic Reviews 2004;(2):CD003946.
[17] Bianchetti A, Scuratti A, Zanetti O, et al. Predictors of mortality and institutionalization in Alzheimer disease patients 1 year after discharge from an Alzheimer dementia unit. Dementia 1995;6(2):108–12.

[18] McCurry SM, Gibbons LE, Logsdon RG, et al. Nighttime insomnia treatment and education for Alzheimer's disease: a randomized, controlled trial. J Am Geriatr Soc 2005; 53(5):793–802.

[19] Shochat T, Martin J, Marler M, et al. Illumination levels in nursing home patients: effects on sleep and activity rhythms. J Sleep Res 2000;9(4):373–9.

[20] Fetveit A, Bjorvatn B. Bright-light treatment reduces actigraphic measured daytime sleep in nursing home patients with dementia. Am J Geriatr Psychiatry 2005;13(5):420–3.

[21] Fetveit A, Bjorvatn B. The effects of bright-light therapy on actigraphical measured sleep last for several weeks post-treatment. A study in a nursing home population. J Sleep Res 2004; 13(2):153–8.

[22] Fetveit A, Skjerve A, Bjorvatn B. Bright light treatment improves sleep in institutionalised elderly—an open trial. Int J Geriatr Psychiatry 2003;18(6):520–6.

[23] Ancoli-Israel S, Martin JL, Kripke DF, et al. Effect of light treatment on sleep and circadian rhythms in demented nursing home patients. J Am Geriatr Soc 2002;50(2):282–9.

[24] Ancoli-Israel S, Gehrman P, Martin JL, et al. Increased light exposure consolidates sleep and strengthens circadian rhythms in severe Alzheimer's disease patients. Behav Sleep Med 2003; 1(1):22–36.

[25] Alessi A, Martin JL, Webber AP, et al. Randomized, controlled trial of a nonpharmacological intervention to improve abnormal sleep/wake patterns in nursing home residents. J Am Geriatr Soc 2005;53(5):803–10.

[26] Ouslander JG, Connell BR, Bliwise DL, et al. A nonpharmacological intervention to improve sleep in nursing home patients: results of a controlled clinical trial. J Am Geriatr Soc 2006;54(1):38–47.

[27] Lyketsos CG, Lindell Veiel L, Baker A, et al. A randomized, controlled trial of bright light therapy for agitated behaviors in dementia patients residing in long-term care. Int J Geriatr Psychiatry 1999;14(7):520–5.

[28] Skjerve A, Holsten F, Aarsland D, et al. Improvement in behavioral symptoms and advance of activity acrophase after short-term bright light treatment in severe dementia. Psychiatry Clin Neurosci 2004;58(4):343–7.

[29] Mishima K, Okawa M, Hishikawa Y, et al. Morning bright light therapy for sleep and behavior disorders in elderly patients with dementia. Acta Psychiatr Scand 1994;89(1):1–7.

[30] Ancoli-Israel S, Martin JL, Gehrman P, et al. Effect of light on agitation in institutionalized patients with severe Alzheimer disease. Am J Geriatr Psychiatry 2003;11(2):194–203.

[31] Eastman CI, Young MA, Fogg LF, et al. Bright light treatment of winter depression: a placebo-controlled trial. Arch Gen Psychiatry 1998;55(10):883–9.

[32] Magnusson A, Kristbjarnarson H. Treatment of seasonal affective disorder with high-intensity light. A phototherapy study with an Icelandic group of patients. J Affect Disord 1991;21(2):141–7.

[33] Joffe RT, Moul DE, Lam RW, et al. Light visor treatment for seasonal affective disorder: a multicenter study. Psychiatry Res 1993;46(1):29–39.

[34] Tuunainen A, Kripke DF, Endo T. Light therapy for non-seasonal depression. Cochrane Depression, Anxiety and Neurosis Group Cochrane Database of Systematic Reviews 2004;(2):CD004050.

[35] Golden RN, Gaynes BN, Ekstrom RD, et al. The efficacy of light therapy in the treatment of mood disorders: a review and meta-analysis of the evidence. Am J Psychiatry 2005;162(4): 656–62.

[36] Tsai YF, Wong TK, Juang YY, et al. The effects of light therapy on depressed elders. Int J Geriatr Psychiatry 2004;19(6):545–8.

[37] Sumaya IC, Rienzi BM, Deegan JF 2nd, et al. Bright light treatment decreases depression in institutionalized older adults: a placebo-controlled crossover study. J Gerontol A Biol Sci Med Sci 2001;56(6):M356–60.

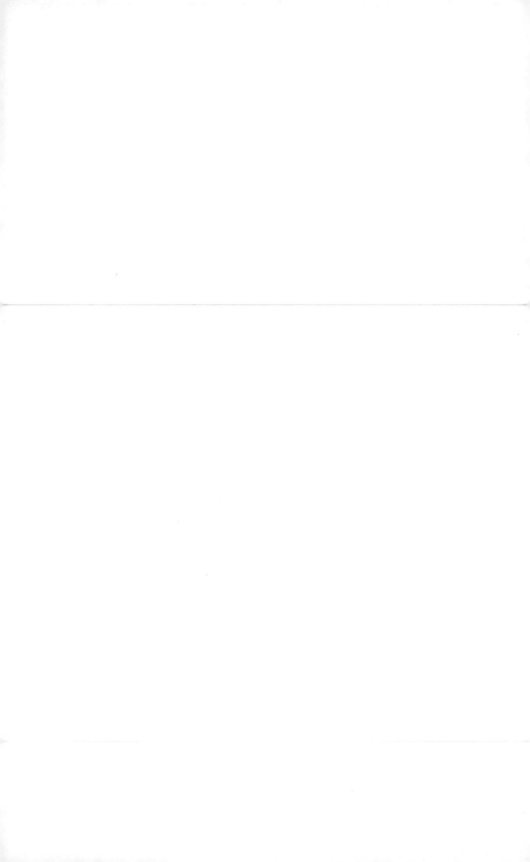

ELSEVIER
SAUNDERS

CLINICS IN
GERIATRIC
MEDICINE

Clin Geriatr Med 24 (2008) 151–165

Obstructive Sleep Apnea in Older Adults

Daniel Norman, MD,
José S. Loredo, MD, MS, MPH, FCCP*

*Division of Pulmonary and Critical Care Medicine,
University of California, San Diego School of Medicine, 9500 Gilman Drive,
MC 0804, San Diego, CA 92093-0804, USA*

Anatomic and physiologic changes that take place during sleep contribute to an environment that predisposes to disordered breathing. Muscles of the oropharynx that normally keep the upper airway patent during wakefulness decrease their tone, especially during rapid eye movement sleep. Supine body position makes it easier for the tongue to fall backward and further narrow the upper airway [1,2]. Behavioral control mechanisms and waking drive to breathe are lost, making respiratory control dependent on the metabolic rate and reduced chemoreceptor responses to carbon dioxide and oxygen, resulting in mild nocturnal hypoventilation [3,4]. A perturbation of any of these anatomic and physiologic changes may result in sleep-disordered breathing. If the airway narrows excessively, then periods of inadequate airflow may occur. Abnormal chemoreceptor responses may result in overcorrection or undercorrection for hypocapnia, hypercapnia, or hypoxemia, causing erratic breathing patterns or periodic breathing and apneas [5].

Obstructive sleep apnea (OSA) occurs when there are recurrent periods of complete or partial upper airway collapse that result in inadequate airflow despite ongoing respiratory muscle effort. Each of these episodes often ends with a transient arousal from sleep (perhaps accompanied by a snort or gasp but rarely a conscious awakening) that results in increased pharyngeal muscle tone and re-establishment of airway patency. When sleep is restored, however, muscle tone wanes and the cycle may repeat; perhaps hundreds of times throughout each night. According to standard definitions, an apnea is a period of cessation (or near cessation) of airflow lasting at least 10 seconds. A hypopnea is a period (lasting at least 10 seconds) of 50% to

---

* Corresponding author. University of California–San Diego Medical Center, 200 W. Arbor Drive, #0804, San Diego, CA 92103-0804.

E-mail address: jloredo@ucsd.edu (J.S. Loredo).

0749-0690/08/$ - see front matter © 2008 Elsevier Inc. All rights reserved.
doi:10.1016/j.cger.2007.08.006   *geriatric.theclinics.com*

90% decline in airflow accompanied by at least a 4% drop in oxyhemoglo-bin saturation or a transient arousal [6]. Many clinicians also recognize periods of diminished airflow that do not last a full 10 seconds, have a de-cline in airflow of less than 50%, or are not accompanied by a 4% decline in oxyhemoglobin saturation, but nonetheless cause obvious disruptions in sleep continuity. These events are termed "respiratory effort–related arousals" [6,7]. Although obstructive events occur when there is upper airway collapse in the setting of ongoing (and often increased) respiratory effort, central events occur when there is a decline in airflow in the setting of a patent airway but diminished or absent respiratory muscle effort. Although they may be seen in anyone, central events are more common in association with certain conditions such as stroke, renal failure, sleeping at high altitude, and congestive heart failure (where, in its most extreme form, they manifest as the respiratory pauses in Cheyne-Stokes respiration) [8]. Mixed events sometimes occur, such as when the upper airway collapses toward the end of a central apnea and remains closed for a time after respi-ratory effort resumes (an obstructive apnea). Whether the events are apneas or hypopneas (central, obstructive, or mixed), OSA not only results in fragmented sleep but also may be accompanied by recurrent transient hypoxemia and dramatic swings in blood pressure and heart rate [9].

To quantify the frequency of these events, sleep clinicians use the terms "apnea hypopnea index" (AHI) to refer to the number of apneas plus the number of hypopneas per hour of sleep, and "respiratory disturbance index" (RDI) to refer to the number of apneas, hypopneas, and respiratory effort–related arousals per hour of sleep. These terms, however, are often used interchangeably. Guidelines vary (and are somewhat arbitrary) with regard to classification of OSA severity, but an AHI between 5 and 19 is typ-ically referred to as mild, an AHI between 20 and 29 as moderate, and an AHI of 30 or more as severe sleep apnea. When the AHI is 5 or higher and associated with excessive daytime somnolence, the patient is diagnosed as having OSA syndrome.

Epidemiology

Among middle-aged adults (30–60 years), the prevalence of OSA (defined as an AHI ≥ 5) is 9% for women and 24% for men, and the prevalence of OSA syndrome (AHI ≥ 5 and daytime hypersomnolence) is 2% for women and 4% for men [10]. In adults older than 60 years, prevalence rates of OSA are considerably higher; often reported in the range of 37.5% to 62% [11,12]. A study of healthy 60-, 70-, and 80-year-olds demonstrated a step-wise increase in the prevalence of sleep-disordered breathing with each decade, such that 2.9% of 60-year-olds, 33.3% of 70-year-olds, and 39.5% of 80-year-olds had an AHI of 5 or higher [13]. In one of the largest epidemiologic studies to date on the subject, the Sleep Heart Health Study evaluated 5615 community-dwelling adults and found a similar stepwise increase in the prevalence of sleep-disordered breathing with advancing age (Fig. 1) [14]. Other investigators have argued that increased prevalence rates of sleep-disordered breathing with age may be largely secondary to increased frequency of central events, and that the prevalence rate of OSA may actually decline after peaking at age 55 years [15]. Epidemiologic data on the prevalence of OSA are further complicated by sex issues. Although middle-aged men are two to three times as likely as premenopausal women to have OSA, the prevalence of OSA increases significantly in postmenopausal women who are not on hormone replacement therapy, approaching the prevalence in men [16]. In a study of 797 premenopausal and 518 postmenopausal women, prevalence of sleep apnea (defined as AHI ≥ 10) was greater in postmenopausal women than premenopausal women (47% versus 21%), and postmenopausal women had a significantly higher mean AHI compared with premenopausal women, even after adjusting for body mass index (BMI) and neck circumference [17].

There is considerable debate regarding why older adults may be at increased risk of OSA. Conditions that are known risk factors for sleep-disordered breathing (such as obesity, diabetes, renal failure, heart disease, hypothyroidism, and stroke) tend to be more common in older adults and may explain part of the increased prevalence in this age group. Obesity is perhaps the most recognized of these risk factors: for every 10-kg increase in additional body weight, the odds ratio for having OSA doubles [10]. One 18-year longitudinal study of older adults supported this notion, suggesting that the changes observed in AHI over time were independent of age and associated only with changes in BMI [18]. In patients who have a history of cerebrovascular accidents, the prevalence rate of sleep-disordered breathing is 62.8% [19]. Diabetes mellitus–associated autonomic neuropathy may alter ventilatory control mechanisms to predispose to the

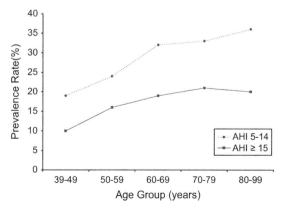

Fig. 1. Prevalence of sleep-disordered breathing by age group. (*Data from* Young T, Shahar E, Nieto FJ, et al. Predictors of sleep-disordered breathing in community-dwelling adults: the Sleep Heart Health Study. Arch Intern Med 2002;162(8):893–900.)

development sleep-disordered breathing [20]. Hypothyroidism is also prevalent in older adults, and increases the risk of OSA [21].

Even in the absence of other comorbid conditions, however, aging itself may be associated with anatomic and physiologic changes that increase the risk of sleep-disordered breathing. Imaging studies have demonstrated that older adults (compared with middle-aged subjects) have changes in bony structure and fat deposits in pharyngeal walls that result in narrower upper airways [22,23]. A few studies, however, have failed to replicate these findings [24,25]. Decreases in pharyngeal dilator muscle activity during sleep are greater in older than in younger adults [26,27], perhaps due to changes in muscle and collagen structure that may take place with age, making airway tissues less rigid. In addition, increasing age is correlated with greater pharyngeal collapsibility, independent of BMI and sex [28,29]. Some studies, but not others, have demonstrated increased airway resistance in older adults compared with younger adults during sleep [26,29–31]. Impaired pharyngeal sensory discrimination in older subjects may also make them more vulnerable to the occurrence and persistence of airway collapse during sleep [32]. Decline in estrogen levels in postmenopausal women may further reduce upper airway muscle activity and increase airway resistance [33–35]. Compared with weight-matched younger adult control subjects, healthy older adults demonstrate wider oscillations in upper airway resistance during supine sleep that may contribute to greater frequency of apneas and hypopneas and a greater tendency for periodic breathing [30]. Older adults also spend a greater percentage of their total sleep time in stage 1 and stage 2 sleep; these stages are marked by greater respiratory instability that may facilitate periodic breathing and tendency to obstruct the upper airway [36,37].

Consequences of obstructive sleep apnea in the general population

In addition to the risks of disrupted sleep and excessive daytime somnolence, OSA has also been associated with increased risk of a multitude of other disorders, affecting a number of different organ systems. To simplify this discussion, these risks are reviewed in two categories: (1) cardiovascular morbidity and mortality and (2) cognitive function and quality of life.

Cardiovascular morbidity and mortality

A number of mechanisms have been proposed whereby OSA may result in increased cardiovascular risk. These mechanisms include increased sympathetic nervous system activity, vascular oxidative stress, endothelial dysfunction, hypercoagulability, insulin resistance, and lately, inflammatory effects from recurrent apnea-associated hypoxemia [38]. Early studies suggested a link between OSA and hypertension, cardiac ischemia, cerebrovascular disease, cardiac arrhythmias, and congestive heart failure but were plagued by questions regarding potential confounding factors [38,39]. Since then, large cross-sectional studies have demonstrated that even after controlling for known confounding factors (such as BMI, neck circumference, age, alcohol consumption, and cigarette smoking), systolic and diastolic blood pressure increase linearly with increasing AHI [40,41]. An observational cohort study of 1022 adults (median follow-up, 3.4 years) found that even after adjustment for age, sex, race, smoking status, alcohol-consumption status, BMI, and the presence or absence of diabetes mellitus, hyperlipidemia, atrial fibrillation, and hypertension, OSA (defined as AHI ≥5) was significantly associated with stroke or death (hazard ratio, 1.97) [42]. Additional studies have demonstrated improvement in cardiac function, reduction in recurrent atrial fibrillation, reduction in blood pressure, and decrease in mortality following treatment of OSA, suggesting a cause-and-effect relationship between sleep-disordered breathing and these disorders [38,43].

Cognitive function and quality of life

Excessive daytime sleepiness is a prominent feature of OSA but not the only cognitive manifestation of this disorder. Compared with controls, apneics demonstrate impaired psychomotor vigilance, accuracy, sustained attention, visuospatial learning, executive function, motor performance, and constructional abilities [44,45]. After 15 days of OSA therapy, however, attention, visuospatial learning, and motor performances return to normal levels [44]. The risk of motor vehicle accidents in OSA increases in a stepwise fashion with increasing apnea severity, such that patients who have moderate to severe OSA have a 15-fold higher rate of accidents than control subjects [46]. Before OSA therapy, apneics demonstrate longer reaction times, divided attention deficits, and twice the number of collisions on driving stimulator tests compared with nonapneic controls; these deficits normalize following continuous positive airway pressure (CPAP) therapy [47]. In neurocognitive testing, apneics demonstrate attention and concentration difficulties, and OSA therapy has resulted in improvements in cognitive function (particularly in attention and vigilance domains) [48]. A recent systematic review of 26 studies concluded that CPAP therapy has a significant positive impact not only on subjective sleepiness but also on depression, fatigue, and general health-related quality of life [49].

Consequences of obstructive sleep apnea in older adults

Cardiovascular morbidity and mortality

Although the cardiovascular consequences of OSA have been well established in the general population, they have been less clearly delineated in older adults. Several studies of older adults have shown an association between OSA and risk of ischemic stroke. In a 6-year longitudinal study of 394 community-dwelling adults 70 to 100 years old, the presence of an AHI 30 or higher significantly increased the risk for subsequent ischemic stroke (hazard ratio, 2.52), even after controlling for all known confounding factors (including age, sex, BMI, blood pressure, cholesterol levels, smoking and alcohol consumption, and the presence or absence of diabetes mellitus, atrial fibrillation, and hypertension) [50]. A study of 51 patients (mean age, 73 years) who had OSA (AHI ≥ 20) who were at least 2 months post ischemic stroke found that those who did not tolerate CPAP therapy were far more likely (36%) to have another vascular event within the ensuing 18 months compared with those who tolerated CPAP therapy (6.7%). Although this trial was not randomized, the authors found that even after adjusting for other vascular risk factors and neurologic indices, the apneics who were tolerant of CPAP were five times less likely to have another vascular event than those who were not tolerant of CPAP [51]. Studies on the effects of OSA on mortality in older adults, however, have yielded mixed or negative findings [52,53]. In a longitudinal study (median follow-up, 4.6 years) of 14,589 men aged 20 to 93 years referred to sleep clinics with suspected sleep apnea, the presence of moderate to severe sleep apnea (AHI > 30) in men younger than 50 years was associated with a relative mortality rate above age-specific rates in the general population [54]. Men aged 50 to 79 years had relative mortality rates close to those of the general population, and men 80 years or older had mortality rates significantly higher than the general population (relative mortality rate, 1.92) [54]. Although there was a similar increase in relative mortality in the subgroup of patients who had the most severe sleep apnea (RDI > 50) and were younger than 50 years, this increase in mortality was not seen in those older than 50 years [54]. A study that examined 233 nursing home patients found a strong association between AHI and mortality in women but not in men [55]. Another longitudinal study of 426 older adults (mean age, 72.5 years) found significantly shorter survival among those who had an AHI of 30 or higher. When adjusted for confounders, however, age, cardiovascular disease, and pulmonary disease (but not AHI) were independent predictors of death [56]. It is not clear why studies to date have failed to find consistent evidence of increased mortality with OSA in older adults. One possible explanation is that mortality in older adults is high enough at baseline that a relatively small increase contributed by OSA is difficult to detect. Some have hypothesized that early mortality in young severe apneics who have cardiovascular risk factors may select patients "resistant" to the deleterious effects of apnea among older subjects [57]. Others have suggested that repetitive transient hypoxemia from apneic events may up-regulate cellular and hormonal mechanisms that protect older OSA patients when later faced with major ischemic events [58]. Further research is needed in this area.

Cognitive function and quality of life

OSA has been associated with daytime sleepiness, poor health, greater limitations in independent activities of daily living, and depression in older adults [12,59]. In older men, higher apnea severity is associated with lower measures of vigilance and executive function [60]. In a cohort of 92 adults between age 50 and 80 years, Phillips and colleagues [61] failed to find significant associations between an AHI of 5 or higher and cognitive function at baseline or at 3-year follow-up [62]. Cohen-Zion and colleagues [63], however, demonstrated that in a cohort of 140 community-dwelling elderly, increases in RDI were associated with decreases in performance on the mini mental status examination over time. Severe sleep-disordered breathing (AHI ≥ 30) in older adults is often associated with impaired attention, memory, executive function, and sequential thinking and planning, but milder forms may only cause cognitive impairment in the presence of excessive daytime sleepiness [64]. One study found that greater AHI negatively impacted memory function in APOE-4 gene carriers, but not in noncarriers [65]. CPAP use in older adults is associated not only with improvements in daytime sleepiness but also with attention, psychomotor speed, executive functioning, and nonverbal delayed recall [64,66]. Stroke patients who also have OSA have greater functional impairment at admission to a rehabilitation unit and at discharge, in addition to 40% longer hospital stays compared with their nonapneic counterparts [67]. To the authors' knowledge, no studies have been performed to date to evaluate risk of motor vehicle accidents in older adults who have OSA. Given the data on excessive daytime somnolence and cognitive deficits with OSA, one might assume that older adults would also be at increased risk. In addition, a number of studies describe an association between OSA and nocturia. In older adults, nocturia increases in frequency with apnea severity, and declines following treatment of OSA [68,69]. It is possible that a combination of frequent nocturia and somnolence in elderly OSA patients could result in increased risk for falls, but specific data are lacking at this time.

Diagnosis

Symptoms and signs

In the general population, typical symptoms that may suggest sleep apnea include loud snoring, gasping arousals from sleep, witnessed apneas, excessive daytime somnolence, night sweats, nonrestorative sleep, and dry mouth or headaches on awakening. Male sex, alcohol consumption, cigarette smoking, and disorders such as hypertension, obesity, diabetes mellitus, renal failure, stroke, heart failure, and atrial fibrillation are known to increase the risk of sleep-disordered breathing and heighten the index of suspicion for the possible presence of OSA. Physical signs that suggest increased risk include truncal obesity (as evidenced by elevated waist-to-hip ratio or a neck circumference > 17 inches in men or > 15 inches in women), palatal ptosis, tonsillar hypertrophy, retrognathia, micrognathia, macroglossia, or other conditions that cause crowding of the oropharynx. Those who have a family history of OSA are also at increased risk [70]. In older adults, some of these signs and symptoms (such as nonrestful sleep, excessive daytime somnolence, and nocturia) may be present, but others (such as such as loud snoring, elevated BMI, and large neck circumference) may not be significantly associated with OSA [71]. Data from the Sleep Heart Health Study on people aged 40 to 98 years demonstrated that male sex, age, BMI, neck girth, snoring, and repeated breathing-pause frequency were associated with OSA, but that as age increased, the magnitude of associations for sleep-disordered breathing and snoring, body habitus, and breathing pauses decreased [72]. Furthermore, some have suggested that older people who have OSA may be less likely to seek medical attention or have the disorder recognized because symptoms of sleepiness, fatigue, morning headache, unintentional napping, concentration difficulties, and so forth may be ascribed to aging itself or to other disorders [73]. Obtaining a careful history and maintaining a high index of suspicion may thus be assets in making the diagnosis.

Diagnostic tests

Overnight attended polysomnography is currently the "gold standard" for the diagnosis of OSA and other forms of sleep-disordered breathing. A full overnight attended polysomnogram usually involves (1) administration of an ECG, an electroencephalogram (EEG), an electrooculogram (EOG), and an electromyogram (EMG) of the chin and anterior tibialis muscles (the latter to detect leg movement during sleep); and (2) measurement of pulse oximetry, airflow (by way of a nasal cannula pressure transducer), respiratory effort, body position, and snoring intensity (using a microphone). Instead of a nasal cannula pressure transducer, some sleep laboratories use a thermistor (a temperature sensor placed between the nostrils and upper lip) to detect airflow, but this method is less sensitive and has fallen out of favor [74]. More limited tests, including portable home studies (often without EEG, EMG, or EOG data) and even simple overnight oximetry, may have a limited role in screening for sleep-disordered breathing in certain high-risk populations [75]. These tests, however, lack valuable data found in the full studies, have not been as extensively studied, and may underestimate apnea severity because they do not provide accurate estimation of the total sleep time.

Treatment of obstructive sleep apnea

Conservative medical management

There is little research focused on older adults on the efficacy of medical management of OSA. All overweight OSA patients should be counseled regarding weight loss; when successful, it can be effective in mitigating (or in some cases, curing) sleep-disordered breathing [76]. Weight-loss medications may be considered; in middle-aged patients, they have demonstrated ability to facilitate weight loss and decrease AHI and symptoms of daytime sleepiness [77]. In older adults, one must be especially cautious regarding side effects and potential drug interactions. Another conservative measure that may help (particularly in cases of positional OSA) is the avoidance of supine positioning during sleep. If tolerated, the "tennis ball technique" (inserting a tennis ball into a pocket sewn to the back of a patient's pajama top adjacent to the lumbar region, thereby making it uncomfortable to lie supine) may be used to facilitate this effort. This technique has been demonstrated in OSA patients not only to improve sleep apnea symptoms but also to reduce blood pressure [78]. Alcohol consumption increases the risk of OSA [79], and its use (particularly near bedtime) should be discouraged. Hypothyroidism (perhaps through weight gain, increased airway edema from myxedema, or other mechanisms) can predispose individuals to OSA [21] and, if present, thyroid replacement therapy can reduce apnea severity [80]. Estrogen use in postmenopausal women may improve sleep-disordered breathing [60]; however, its routine use for improving OSA cannot be recommended in light of its risks of serious cardiovascular sequelae.

Continuous positive airway pressure therapy

CPAP is considered the gold standard in the treatment of OSA. In CPAP therapy, patients wear a snug-fitting mask over their nose (or nose and mouth) that is connected by way of a hose to a bedside device that delivers airflow under pressure during sleep. The air pressure the unit delivers is determined during polysomnography (a CPAP titration study) or by computer algorithms in autotitrating CPAP machines, to act as a pneumatic splint to keep the upper airway patent. CPAP therapy can lessen daytime sleepiness [66], improve some measures of cognitive function [64], and diminish frequency of nocturia in older adults who have OSA [81]. Although CPAP therapy may be difficult for some to tolerate, patient education about OSA and the benefits of CPAP, in addition to evaluation of obstacles encountered during CPAP therapy, can improve compliance in older adults [82]. A retrospective review of 44 older adults who had OSA (baseline AHI, 37.6) found a stepwise decrease in CPAP compliance with increase in age. Twenty-three percent of 55- to 59-year-olds, 27% of 60- to 64-year-olds, 33% of 65- to 70-year-olds, and 42% of those 70 years and older were noncompliant with CPAP therapy. These data should be interpreted with caution, however, because the oldest group was also the group with the lowest baseline AHI (26.6 versus 37.6 for group as whole) [83]. The ability to tolerate CPAP therapy in stroke patients varies according to different studies, from 12% to 70% [84–86], and some have suggested that the benefits of CPAP therapy in improving functional outcomes might be limited in this population of patients [87]. In a recent study, patients who had

Alzheimer's disease and OSA tolerated CPAP treatment well [66]; therefore, poor cognitive function should not preclude an older adult who has OSA from a trial of CPAP therapy. Compliant use of CPAP in older adults was associated with improvement in attention, psychomotor speed, executive functioning, and nonverbal delayed recall. Surprisingly, those who were the least vigilant at baseline were more likely to comply with treatment [64].

Oral appliance therapy

Oral appliances for the treatment of sleep-disordered breathing are fitted by specialty dentists and worn at night to enhance airway patency by moving the mandible or tongue forward. Although CPAP is considered first-line therapy and more effective at reducing AHI, oral appliances have also been shown to reduce daytime sleepiness and decrease blood pressure in OSA patients [88–90]. Predictors of efficacy include milder OSA severity, positional sleep apnea (higher AHI in the supine versus the lateral sleep position), lower BMI, and greater ability to protrude the mandible [88]. Possible side effects include temporomandibular joint pain, drooling during sleep, tooth pain, and tooth movement resulting in malocclusion [88]. Currently, no studies have assessed oral appliance use specifically in older adults, but one study suggested a better treatment response in younger patients [91]. In addition, older adults who have poor dentition may not be candidates for oral appliance therapy, for obvious reasons.

Surgery

Options for surgical therapy for OSA generally fall into one of five categories: (1) techniques designed to widen the oropharynx and hypopharynx, (2) nasal reconstructive surgery, (3) maxillary-mandibular advancement surgery, (4) tracheotomy, and (5) bariatric surgery (Box 1). A recent meta-analysis reported that only 31.5% of uvulopalatopharyngoplasty surgeries reduce the AHI to lower than 10 and only 13% result in an AHI of 5 or lower. Maxillary-mandibular advancement surgery has a somewhat better success rate, with 45% and 43% resulting in an AHI of 10 or lower and an AHI of 5 or lower, respectively [92]. In light of these findings, some have suggested that current evidence does not support the use of surgery in sleep apnea [88]. Careful consideration of the potential risks and benefits of surgery should be undertaken before recommending it to any older adult who has OSA. Adenotonsillectomy is useful in the treatment of OSA in children but are rarely used in adults, in whom tonsillar hypertrophy is less common and plays a minor role in airway obstruction. Nasal surgeries are rarely successful in improving OSA severity [93]; however, surgical correction of partial nasal obstruction may improve CPAP tolerance [94]. There is a paucity of data regarding the efficacy of the other categories of surgical techniques for OSA (see Box 1), and the authors are not aware of any studies that focus specifically on surgical therapy for OSA in the older adult.

Box 1. Surgical modalities for treatment of obstructive sleep apnea

Techniques designed to widen the oropharynx and hypopharynx
- Uvulopalatopharyngoplasty
- Genioglossal advancement
- Hyoid bone suspension
- Laser-assisted uvulopalatoplasty
- Adenotonsillectomy
- Lingualplasty
- Somnoplasty (radiofrequency volumetric reduction)
- Pillar procedure implants

Nasal reconstructive surgery
- Turbinate reduction
- Septoplasty
- Somnoplasty

Maxillary-mandibular advancement surgery
Tracheotomy
Bariatric surgery

Tracheotomy can cure the most severe cases of OSA because it completely bypasses the sites of upper airway obstruction; however, given its high morbidity and the availability of other treatment options, tracheotomy is often considered a "last resort" procedure for the treatment of severe, life-threatening OSA unresponsive to other treatment modalities. Bariatric surgery can be a helpful adjunct to the treatment of morbidly obese patients who have OSA, often resulting in significant improvement in OSA severity [91].

Summary

OSA represents the most severe stage of the spectrum of sleep-disordered breathing. OSA presents with symptoms of chronic loud snoring and daytime sleepiness. In middle-aged adults, OSA increases the risks of cardiovascular morbidity, mortality, cognitive dysfunction, and reduced quality of life. Although OSA is likely to be more prevalent in the older adult, less is known about its sequelae in this age group. There are no convincing data at this time that OSA in older adults independently increases mortality, but several studies show an association between OSA and increased daytime sleepiness, cognitive dysfunction, nocturia, and reduced quality of life. A high index of suspicion, careful clinical history, and appropriate sleep testing is necessary for the diagnosis of OSA in the older adult because the symptoms of OSA are often attributed to the process of aging itself by the patient and by the medical provider. Among therapeutic options,

CPAP is the most effective modality used to treat OSA in the older adult and is generally well tolerated, even in the setting of cognitive impairment.

References

[1] Horner RL, Shea SA, McIvor J, et al. Pharyngeal size and shape during wakefulness and sleep in patients with obstructive sleep apnoea. Q J Med 1989;72(268):719–35.

[2] Tsuiki S, Almeida FR, Bhalla PS, et al. Supine-dependent changes in upper airway size in awake obstructive sleep apnea patients. Sleep Breath 2003;7(1):43–50.

[3] Skatrud JB, Dempsey JA. Interaction of sleep state and chemical stimuli in sustaining rhythmic ventilation. J Appl Physiol 1983;55(3):813–22.

[4] Mahamed S, Hanly PJ, Babor J, et al. Overnight changes of chemoreflex control in obstructive sleep apnoea patients. Respir Physiol Neurobiol 2005;146(2–3):279–90.

[5] Younes M, Ostrowski M, Thompson W, et al. Chemical control stability in patients with obstructive sleep apnea. Am J Respir Crit Care Med 2001;163(5):1181–90.

[6] Sleep-related breathing disorders in adults: recommendations for syndrome definition and measurement techniques in clinical research. The Report of an American Academy of Sleep Medicine Task Force. Sleep 1999;22(5):667–89.

[7] Guilleminault C, Stoohs R, Clerk A, et al. A cause of excessive daytime sleepiness. The upper airway resistance syndrome. Chest 1993;104(3):781–7.

[8] De Backer WA. Central sleep apneoea, pathogenesis and treatment: an overview and perspective. Eur Respir J 1995;8:1372–83.

[9] Somers VK, Dyken ME, Clary MP, et al. Sympathetic neural mechanisms in obstructive sleep apnea. J Clin Invest 1995;96(4):1897–904.

[10] Young T, Palta M, Dempsey J, et al. The occurrence of sleep-disordered breathing among middle-aged adults. N Engl J Med 1993;328:1230–5.

[11] Ancoli-Israel S, Kripke DF, Mason W, et al. Sleep apnea and nocturnal myoclonus in a senior population. Sleep 1981;4(4):349–58.

[12] Ancoli-Israel S, Kripke DF, Klauber MR, et al. Sleep-disordered breathing in community-dwelling elderly. Sleep 1991;14:486–95.

[13] Hoch CC, Reynolds CF 3rd, Monk TH, et al. Comparison of sleep-disordered breathing among healthy elderly in the seventh, eighth, and ninth decades of life. Sleep 1990;13:502–11.

[14] Young T, Shahar E, Nieto FJ, et al. Predictors of sleep-disordered breathing in community-dwelling adults: the Sleep Heart Health Study. Arch Intern Med 2002;162(8):893–900.

[15] Bixler EO, Vgontzas AN, Ten Have T, et al. Effects of age on sleep apnea in men. I. Prevalence and severity. Am J Respir Crit Care Med 1998;157(1):144–8.

[16] Bixler EO, Vgontzas AN, Lin HM, et al. Prevalence of sleep-disordered breathing in women: effects of gender. Am J Respir Crit Care Med 2001;163(3 Pt 1):608–13.

[17] Dancey DR, Hanly PJ, Soong C, et al. Impact of menopause on the prevalence and severity of sleep apnea. Chest 2001;120(1):151–5.

[18] Ancoli-Israel S, Gehrman P, Kripke DF, et al. Long-term follow-up of sleep disordered breathing in older adults. Sleep Med 2001;2(6):511–6.

[19] Wierzbicka A, Rola R, Wichniak A, et al. The incidence of sleep apnea in patients with stroke or transient ischemic attack. J Physiol Pharmacol 2006;57(4):385–90.

[20] Peltier AC, Consens FB, Sheikh K, et al. Autonomic dysfunction in obstructive sleep apnea is associated with impaired glucose regulation. Sleep Med 2007;8(2):149–55.

[21] Skjodt NM, Atkar R, Easton PA. Screening for hypothyroidism in sleep apnoea. Am J Respir Crit Care Med 1999;160:732–5.

[22] Martin SE, Mathur R, Marshall I, et al. The effect of age, sex, obesity and posture on upper airway size. Eur Respir J 1997;10:2087–90.

[23] Malhotra A, Huang Y, Fogel R, et al. Aging influences on pharyngeal anatomy and physiology: the predisposition to pharyngeal collapse. Am J Med 2006;119(1):72.e9–14.

[24] Burger CD, Stanson AW, Sheedy PF 2nd, et al. Fast-computed tomography evaluation of age-related changes in upper airway structure and function in normal men. Am Rev Respir Dis 1992;145:846–52.

[25] Mayer P, Pepin JL, Bettega G, et al. Relationship between body mass index, age and upper airway measurements in snorers and sleep apnoea patients. Eur Respir J 1996;9:1801–9.

[26] Worsnop C, Kay A, Kim Y, et al. Effect of age on sleep onset-related changes in respiratory pump and upper airway muscle function. J Appl Physiol 2000;88(5):1831–9.

[27] Crow HC, Ship JA. Tongue strength and endurance in different aged individuals. J Gerontol A Biol Sci Med Sci 1996;51:M247–50.

[28] Fogel RB, White DP, Pierce RJ, et al. Control of upper airway muscle activity in younger versus older men during sleep onset. J Physiol 2003;553(Pt 2):533–44.

[29] Eikermann M, Jordan AS, Chamberlin NL, et al. The influence of aging on pharyngeal collapsibility during sleep. Chest 2007;131(6):1702–9.

[30] Hudgel DW, Devadatta P, Hamilton H. Pattern of breathing and upper airway mechanics during wakefulness and sleep in healthy elderly humans. J Appl Physiol 1993;74:2198–204.

[31] Thurnheer R, Wraith PK, Douglas NJ. Influence of age and gender on upper airway resistance in NREM and REM sleep. J Appl Physiol 2001;90:981–8.

[32] Aviv JE, Martin JH, Jones ME, et al. Age-related changes in pharyngeal and supraglottic sensation. Ann Otol Rhinol Laryngol 1994;103:749–52.

[33] Popovic RM, White DP. Upper airway muscle activity in normal women: influence of hormonal status. J Appl Physiol 1998;84(3):1055–62.

[34] Saaresranta T, Polo-Kantola P, Rauhala E, et al. Medroxyprogesterone in postmenopausal females with partial upper airway obstruction during sleep. Eur Respir J 2001;18:989–95.

[35] Driver HS, McLean H, Kumar DV, et al. The influence of the menstrual cycle on upper airway resistance and breathing during sleep. Sleep 2005;28:449–56.

[36] Trinder J, Whitworth F, Kay A, et al. Respiratory instability during sleep onset. J Appl Physiol 1992;73:2462–9.

[37] Ohayon MM, Carskadon MA, Guilleminault C, et al. Meta-analysis of quantitative sleep parameters from childhood to old age in healthy individuals: developing normative sleep values across the human lifespan. Sleep 2004;27:1255–73.

[38] Shamsuzzaman AS, Gersh BJ, Somers VK. Obstructive sleep apnea: implications for cardiac and vascular disease. JAMA 2003;290(14):1906–14.

[39] Wolk R, Somers VK. Cardiovascular consequences of obstructive sleep apnea. Clin Chest Med 2003;24(2):195–205.

[40] Young T, Peppard P, Palta M, et al. Population-based study of sleep-disordered breathing as a risk factor for hypertension. Arch Intern Med 1997;157(15):1746–52.

[41] Nieto FJ, Young TB, Lind BK, et al. Association of sleep-disordered breathing, sleep apnea, and hypertension in a large community-based study. Sleep Heart Health Study. JAMA 2000; 283(14):1829–36.

[42] Yaggi HK, Concato J, Kernan WN, et al. Obstructive sleep apnea as a risk factor for stroke and death. N Engl J Med 2005;353(19):2034–41.

[43] Doherty LS, Kiely JL, Swan V, et al. Long-term effects of nasal continuous positive airway pressure therapy on cardiovascular outcomes in sleep apnea syndrome. Chest 2005;127(6): 2076–84.

[44] Ferini-Strambi L, Baietto C, Di Gioia MR, et al. Cognitive dysfunction in patients with obstructive sleep apnea (OSA): partial reversibility after continuous positive airway pressure (CPAP). Brain Res Bull 2003;61(1):87–92.

[45] Sforza E, Haba-Rubio J, De Bilbao F, et al. Performance vigilance task and sleepiness in patients with sleep-disordered breathing. Eur Respir J 2004;24(2):279–85.

[46] Horstmann S, Hess CW, Bassetti C, et al. Sleepiness-related accidents in sleep apnea patients. Sleep 2000;23(3):383–9.

[47] Mazza S, Pepin JL, Naegele B, et al. Driving ability in sleep apnoea patients before and after CPAP treatment: evaluation on a road safety platform. Eur Respir J 2006;28(5):1020–8.

[48] Aloia MS, Arnedt JT, Davis JD, et al. Neuropsychological sequelae of obstructive sleep apnea-hypopnea syndrome: a critical review. J Int Neuropsychol Soc 2004;10(5):772–85.

[49] McMahon JP, Foresman BH, Chisholm RC. The influence of CPAP on the neurobehavioral performance of patients with obstructive sleep apnea hypopnea syndrome: a systematic review. WMJ 2003;102(1):36–43.

[50] Munoz R, Duran-Cantolla J, Martinez-Vila E, et al. Severe sleep apnea and risk of ischemic stroke in the elderly. Stroke 2006;37(9):2317–21.

[51] Martinez-Garcia MA, Galiano-Blancart R, Roman-Sanchez P, et al. Continuous positive airway pressure treatment in sleep apnea prevents new vascular events after ischemic stroke. Chest 2005;128(4):2123–9.

[52] Mant A, King M, Saunders NA, et al. Four-year follow-up of mortality and sleep-related respiratory disturbance in non-demented seniors. Sleep 1995;18:433–8.

[53] He J, Kryger MH, Zorick FJ, et al. Mortality and apnea index in obstructive sleep apnea. Chest 1988;94:9–14.

[54] Lavie P, Herer P, Peled R, et al. Mortality in sleep apnea patients: a multivariate analysis of risk factors. Sleep 1995;18:149–57.

[55] Ancoli-Israel S, Klauber MR, Kripke DF, et al. Sleep apnea in female patients in a nursing home. Increased risk of mortality. Chest 1989;96(5):1054–8.

[56] Ancoli-Israel S, Kripke D, Klauber M, et al. Morbidity, mortality and sleep-disordered breathing in community dwelling elderly. Sleep 1996;19:277–82.

[57] Launois SH, Pepin JL, Levy P. Sleep apnea in the elderly: a specific entity? Sleep Med Rev 2007;11(2):87–97.

[58] Lavie L, Lavie P. Ischemic preconditioning as a possible explanation for the age decline relative mortality in sleep apnea. Med Hypotheses 2006;66(6):1069–73.

[59] Enright PL, Newman AB, Wahl PW, et al. Prevalence and correlates of snoring and observed apneas in 5201 older adults. Sleep 1996;19:531–8.

[60] Saaresranta T, Polo-Kantola P, Virtanen I, et al. Menopausal estrogen therapy predicts better nocturnal oxyhemoglobin saturation. Maturitas 2006;55(3):255–63.

[61] Phillips B, Berry D, Schmitt F, et al. Sleep-disordered breathing in the healthy elderly. Chest 1992;101:345–9.

[62] Phillips B, Berry D, Schmitt F, et al. Sleep-disordered breathing in healthy aged persons: two- and three-year follow-up. Sleep 1994;17:411–5.

[63] Cohen-Zion M, Stepnowsky C, Johnson S, et al. Cognitive changes and sleep disordered breathing in elderly: differences in race. J Psychosom Res 2004;56(5):549–53.

[64] Aloia MS, Ilniczky N, Di Dio P, et al. Neuropsychological changes and treatment compliance in older adults with sleep apnea. J Psychosom Res 2003;54(1):71–6.

[65] O'Hara R, Schröder CM, Kraemer HC, et al. Nocturnal sleep apnea/hypopnea is associated with lower memory performance in APOE epsilon4 carriers. Neurology 2005; 65(4):642–4.

[66] Chong MS, Ayalon L, Marler M, et al. Continuous positive airway pressure reduces subjective daytime sleepiness in patients with mild to moderate Alzheimer's disease with sleep disordered breathing. J Am Geriatr Soc 2006;54(5):777–81.

[67] Kaneko Y, Hajek VE, Zivanovic V, et al. Relationship of sleep apnea to functional capacity and length of hospitalization following stroke. Sleep 2003;26:293–7.

[68] Fitzgerald MP, Mulligan M, Parthasarathy S. Nocturic frequency is related to severity of obstructive sleep apnea, improves with continuous positive airways treatment. Am J Obstet Gynecol 2006;194(5):1399–403.

[69] Endeshaw YW, Johnson TM, Kutner MH, et al. Sleep-disordered breathing and nocturia in older adults. J Am Geriatr Soc 2004;52(6):957–60.

[70] Kaparianos A, Sampsonas F, Karkoulias K, et al. Obstructive sleep apnoea syndrome and genes. Neth J Med 2006;64(8):280–9.

[71] Endeshaw Y. Clinical characteristics of obstructive sleep apnea in community-dwelling older adults. J Am Geriatr Soc 2006;54(11):1740–4.

[72] Cohen-Zion M, Stepnowsky C, Marler T, et al. Changes in cognitive function associated with sleep disordered breathing in older people. J Am Geriatr Soc 2001;49(12):1622–7.

[73] Groth M. Sleep apnea in the elderly. Clin Geriatr Med 2005;21:701–12.

[74] Norman RG, Ahmed MM, Walsleben JA, et al. Detection of respiratory events during NPSG: nasal cannula/pressure sensor versus thermistor. Sleep 1997;20(12):1175–84.

[75] Flemons WW, Littner MR, Rowley JA, et al. Home diagnosis of sleep apnea: a systematic review of the literature. An evidence review cosponsored by the American Academy of Sleep Medicine, the American College of Chest Physicians, and the American Thoracic Society. Chest 2003;124(4):1543–79.

[76] Peppard PE, Young T, Palta M, et al. Longitudinal study of moderate weight change and sleep-disordered breathing. JAMA 2000;284(23):3015–21.

[77] Yee BJ, Phillips CL, Banerjee D, et al. The effect of sibutramine-assisted weight loss in men with obstructive sleep apnoea. Int J Obes (Lond) 2007;31(1):161–8.

[78] Berger M, Oksenberg A, Silverberg DS, et al. Avoiding the supine position during sleep lowers 24 h blood pressure in obstructive sleep apnea (OSA) patients. J Hum Hypertens 1997;11(10):657–64.

[79] Peppard PE, Austin D, Brown RL. Association of alcohol consumption and sleep disordered breathing in men and women. J Clin Sleep Med 2007;3(3):265–70.

[80] Rajagopal KR, Abbrecht PH, Derderian SS, et al. Obstructive sleep apnea in hypothyroidism. Ann Intern Med 1984;101(4):491–4.

[81] Weaver TE, Chasens ER. Continuous positive airway pressure treatment for sleep apnea in older adults. Sleep Med Rev 2007;11:99–111.

[82] Aloia MS, Dio LD, Ilniczky N, et al. Improving compliance with nasal CPAP and vigilance in older adults with OSAHS. Sleep Breath 2001;5(1):13–22.

[83] Doerr C, Mcleland J, Kampelman J, et al. Objective CPAP compliance in the older adult population. Sleep 2007;30:A183.

[84] Hui DS, Choy DK, Wong LK, et al. Prevalence of sleep-disordered breathing and continuous positive airway pressure compliance: results in Chinese patients with first-ever ischemic stroke. Chest 2002;122:852–60.

[85] Sandberg O, Franklin KA, Bucht G, et al. Nasal continuous positive airway pressure in stroke patients with sleep apnoea: a randomized treatment study. Eur Respir J 2001;18:630–4.

[86] Wessendorf TE, Wang YM, Thilmann AF, et al. Treatment of obstructive sleep apnoea with nasal continuous positive airway pressure in stroke. Eur Respir J 2001;18:623–9.

[87] Hsu CY, Vennelle M, Li HY, et al. Sleep-disordered breathing after stroke: a randomised controlled trial of continuous positive airway pressure. J Neurol Neurosurg Psychiatry 2006;77(10):1143–9.

[88] Sundaram S, Bridgman SA, Lim J, et al. Surgery for obstructive sleep apnoea. Cochrane Database Syst Rev 2005;(4):CD001004.

[89] Otsuka R, Ribeiro de Almeida F, Lowe AA, et al. The effect of oral appliance therapy on blood pressure in patients with obstructive sleep apnea. Sleep Breath 2006;10(1):29–36.

[90] Gotsopoulos H, Kelly JJ, Cistulli PA. Oral appliance therapy reduces blood pressure in obstructive sleep apnea: a randomized, controlled trial. Sleep 2004;27(5):934–41.

[91] Fritscher LG, Mottin CC, Canani S, et al. Obesity and obstructive sleep apnea-hypopnea syndrome: the impact of bariatric surgery. Obes Surg 2007;17(1):95–9.

[92] Elshaug AG, Moss JR, Southcott A, et al. Redefining success in airway surgery for obstructive sleep apnea: a meta analysis and synthesis of the evidence. Sleep 2007;30(4):461–7.

[93] Series F, St Pierre S, Carrier G. Effects of surgical correction of nasal obstruction in the treatment of obstructive sleep apnea. Am Rev Respir Dis 1992;146(5 Pt 1):1261–5.

[94] Powell NB, Zonato AI, Weaver EM, et al. Radiofrequency treatment of turbinate hypertrophy in subjects using continuous positive airway pressure: a randomized, double-blind, placebo-controlled clinical pilot trial. Laryngoscope 2001;111(10):1783–90.

ELSEVIER
SAUNDERS

Clin Geriatr Med 24 (2008) 167–180

CLINICS IN
GERIATRIC
MEDICINE

Restless Legs Syndrome in Older Adults

Kai Spiegelhalder, Dipl.-Psych.,
Magdolna Hornyak, MD*

*Sleep Disorders Center, Department of Psychiatry and Psychotherapy,
University Hospital Freiburg, Hauptstrasse 5, D-79104 Freiburg, Germany*

Restless legs syndrome (RLS) is a prevalent disorder in the general population, occurring with increasing frequency and severity in the elderly. RLS symptoms show strong circadian rhythmicity, with a peak of symptom severity between midnight and 3 AM; as a consequence of this, most patients complain about sleep disturbances. Although RLS symptoms are common in the general population, many patients with RLS are still unrecognized or misdiagnosed. This has lead to RLS being referred to as "the most common disorder you never heard of." A survey conducted from 2002 to 2003 in North America found that general physicians only meet the correct diagnosis of RLS in less than 10% of cases [1]. Given that the diagnosis of RLS is a clinical diagnosis, the level of underdiagnosis may well be more pronounced in the elderly, especially people who are less able to express their complaints in as detailed and clear a fashion as the general adult population might. The inappropriate treatment of RLS, such as in the use of antidepressants or neuroleptics for nighttime sedation, can aggravate RLS symptoms. A recently published study found age, number of comorbidities, number of physician visits, and use of (presumably inappropriate) prescription medications to negatively impact on health-related quality of life in RLS [2]. The accurate diagnosis and therapy of the disorder is therefore essential, and can substantially improve the quality of sleep and life in this patient population. This article attempts to give a summary of the recent knowledge on diagnosis, epidemiology, and treatment of RLS in the elderly.

Diagnosis criteria of restless legs syndrome

Restless legs syndrome typically presents with an urge to move the legs. The urge to move is usually accompanied by unpleasant sensations. Many

* Corresponding author.
E-mail address: magdolna.hornyak@uniklinik-freiburg.de (M. Hornyak).

0749-0690/08/$ - see front matter © 2008 Elsevier Inc. All rights reserved.
doi:10.1016/j.cger.2007.08.004
geriatric.theclinics.com

patients encounter difficulties in describing the sensations except to say that they are uncomfortable and deep inside the legs, while other patients report sensations like "tearing," "burning," "electric current," or "painful." A prominent feature of the disorder is the circadian rhythmicity of the symptoms, with onset or increase in the evening or at night. With disease progression, some patients also develop symptoms during the day and in other parts of the body, most often in the arms. RLS symptoms improve by moving the affected limb and worsen with rest. Clinically, the diagnosis of RLS is based on the patient's description. Diagnostic criteria and clinical characteristics of the disorder were outlined in 1995 [3] and newly revised [4]. Diagnostic criteria are summarized in Box 1.

Because of the nocturnal appearance of symptoms, RLS has high impact on sleep. Sleep disturbances are the most frequent reason for the patients to seek medical aid. In polysomnographic studies, subjects with RLS display considerably disrupted sleep [5] and 80% to 90% of subjects reveal an elevated number of periodic leg movements during sleep (PLMS) [6]. PLMS are a sleep phenomenon with periodic episodes of repetitive stereotyped leg movements [7,8] and are characterized by the extension of the big toe in combination with flexion of the ankle, knee, and sometimes the hip. The muscle that is most frequently involved in PLMS is the tibialis anterior muscle [9]. A PLMS index (number of PLMS per hour of sleep) greater than 10 is considered pathologic [10]. Most RLS patients also show periodic leg movements in polysomnographic recordings while awake [6]. PLMS may also frequently occur in other sleep disorders [11], such as narcolepsy [12,13], sleep apnea syndrome [14], or rapid eye movement sleep behavior disorder [15]. In the elderly, PLMS have also been frequently observed in subjects without any sleep disturbance [16].

Diagnosis of restless legs syndrome in the elderly

The diagnosis of RLS is based on the patient's history. The ability to verbally express experienced bodily sensations may be diminished in the elderly by the impact of comorbid conditions, such as cognitive impairment, speech disorders, or aphasic syndromes, while cognitive deficits might be induced or exacerbated by the restless legs syndrome itself [17]. This has lead to the proposal for a modification of diagnostic criteria in this special group of patients. The modified criteria emphasize the inclusion of behavioral indicators and supportive features within the diagnostic work-up (Box 2) [4]. The observation of behavior might be helpful for the diagnosis: for instance, rubbing the legs or excessive motor activity during the night may indicate the patient's sensations and the urge to move. A detailed history of family members and of caregivers is considered to be very important in diagnosing RLS in the impaired elderly. Conditions mimicking RLS especially require carefully differentiated consideration in the elderly. Painful states, such as

Box 1. Diagnosis criteria of RLS

Essential criteria[a]
1. An urge to move the legs, usually accompanied or caused by uncomfortable and unpleasant sensations in the legs (Sometimes the urge to move is present without the uncomfortable sensations and sometimes the arms or other body parts are involved in addition to the legs.)
2. The urge to move or unpleasant sensations begin or worsen during periods of rest or inactivity, such as lying or sitting
3. The urge to move or unpleasant sensations are partially or totally relieved by movement, such as walking or stretching, at least as long as the activity continues
4. The urge to move or unpleasant sensations are worse in the evening or night than during the day, or only occur in the evening or night (When symptoms are very severe, the worsening at night may not be noticeable but must have been previously present.)

Supportive criteria
1. Positive family history of RLS
2. Response to dopaminergic therapy
3. Periodic limb movements (during wakefulness or sleep)

Associated criteria
1. Natural clinical course
2. Sleep disturbance
3. Medical evaluation or physical examination

---

[a] All four essential criteria are necessary for the diagnosis, the supportive criteria can help resolve any diagnostic uncertainty.
Adapted from Allen RP, Picchietti D, Hening WA, et al. Restless legs syndrome: diagnostic criteria, special considerations and epidemiology. A report from the restless legs syndrome diagnosis and epidemiology workshop at the National Institute of Health. Sleep Med 2003;4(2):101–19; with permission.

neuropathy, arthrotic conditions involving the lower limbs, or leg cramps may be distinguished from RLS symptoms, as they are not characterized by a circadian rhythm with an increase of severity in the evening or at night. Other differential diagnoses, such as venous insufficiency of the legs, are mostly accompanied with skin manifestations. Neuroleptic induced akathisia can be diagnosed by the typical symptomatology of a continuous urge to move the legs, body-rocking, and drug history. Akathisia is not as focal as RLS, occurs independently of the body's position, and produces milder sleep disturbances [18].

Box 2. Diagnostic criteria for the diagnosis of probable RLS in the cognitively impaired elderly

Essential criteria[a]

1. Signs of leg discomfort, such as rubbing or kneading the legs and groaning while holding the lower extremities
2. Excessive motor activity in the lower extremities, such as pacing, fidgeting, repetitive kicking, tossing and turning in bed, slapping the legs on the mattress, cycling movements of the lower limbs, repetitive foot tapping, rubbing the feet together, and the inability to remain seated
3. Signs of leg discomfort are exclusively present or worsen during periods of rest or inactivity
4. Signs of leg discomfort are diminished with activity
5. Criteria 1 and 2 occur only in the evening or at night, or are worse at those times than during the day

Supportive criteria

1. Dopaminergic responsiveness
2. Patient's past history—as reported by a family member, caregiver or friend—is suggestive of RLS
3. A first degree, biologic relative (sibling, child, or parent) has RLS
4. Observed periodic limb movements while awake or during sleep
5. Periodic limb movements of sleep recorded by polysomnography or actigraphy
6. Significant sleep-onset problems
7. Better quality sleep in the day than at night
8. The use of restraints at night (for institutionalized patients)
9. Low serum ferritin level
10. End-stage renal disease
11. Diabetes
12. Clinical, electromyographic, or nerve-conduction evidence of peripheral neuropathy or radiculopathy

---

[a] According to Allen et al [4], all five essential criteria are necessary for the diagnosis.

Adapted from Allen RP, Picchietti D, Hening WA, et al. Restless legs syndrome: diagnostic criteria, special considerations and epidemiology. A report from the restless legs syndrome diagnosis and epidemiology workshop at the National Institute of Health. Sleep Med 2003;4(2):101–19; with permission.

Prevalence of restless legs syndrome in the elderly

Most patients presenting to physicians with typical RLS symptoms are of middle to older age. However, symptoms often start in childhood and early adolescence [19], beginning in 38% to 45% of the cases before the age of 20, as reported by adult subjects in retrospective studies [6,20]. Usually, the symptoms of RLS are mild in early adulthood and progress with advancing age. A need for treatment mostly starts at the age of 50 or 60 [20].

Population studies suggest two phenotypes of the disease. On the one hand, patients who reported the onset of their symptoms early in life appear to have a significantly higher incidence of affected relatives than those who reported symptom onset later in life [21–24]. These patients are believed to show a low rate of occurrence of small-fiber neuropathy [25] when compared with those at a later age of symptom onset. On the other hand, patients without a positive family history of the disease were reported to have a later age of symptom onset and a higher incidence of neuropathy [26,27]. Changes of iron metabolism and low ferritin levels were found in both early-onset [24,28,29] and late-onset RLS [30,31]. Patients with a later onset of RLS were found in one study to be more likely to complain of insomnia than patients with earlier onset of RLS, the latter tending to report hypersomnic complaints, such as daytime sleepiness [32].

Epidemiologic studies investigating the age distribution of RLS revealed a strong increase in the prevalence in the elderly. The prevalence of two RLS-related complaints in a Canadian survey increased from 9% and 5% (18- to 20-year-old age group) to 23% and 18% (equal to or over 60-year-old age group) over the life-span [33]. Experiencing the symptoms of restless legs for five or more nights per month was found to be significantly associated with increased age in the Kentucky Behavioral Risk Factor Surveillance Survey [34]. The main finding of the survey was a 3% prevalence in participants aged 18 to 29 years, but a prevalence of up to 19% in those 80 years and older. Ulfberg and colleagues [35] found an increase in the prevalence of RLS from 1.2% in the age group 18 to 24 years, to 10.5% in the age group of 55 to 64 years in a questionnaire study in central Sweden. The study of Ohayon and Roth [36] performed with the Sleep-EVAL telephone interview system, indicated a 5.5% prevalence of RLS in 18,980 subjects representative of the general population of five European countries. The study demonstrated a nearly linear increase of the RLS prevalence from 2.7% in the age group 15 to 19 years, up to 8.7% in the age group 70 years and older. Similarly, a population-based survey in which face-to-face interviews were conducted in 10,263 subjects in France showed an overall prevalence of 8.5%, increasing from 5.2% in the age group of 18 to 24 years to 11.3% in the age group of 50 to 64 years [37]. A population-based study conducted in Norway and Denmark [38] found an 11.5% prevalence of RLS, with a significant difference between the age group 18 to 29 years and the older adults. However, no age-related differences were found above the age of 30 years.

No differences in gender were found in the Canadian survey [33], the Kentucky survey [34], and in a community-based study in Wisconsin [39]. However, the Sleep-EVAL study [36] and the French study [37], which have been the largest studies to date, the survey of Bjorvatn and colleagues [38], two German studies [40,41], and an Austrian survey [42], found the prevalence in women to be approximately twice as high as in men. The prevalence in women increases with the number of childbirths [41].

Comorbidity and secondary forms of restless legs syndrome in the elderly

Surveys have found several disorders to be associated with RLS. Furthermore, RLS may manifest as a secondary disorder because of an underlying primary disease. Anemia and terminal renal disease are well-known conditions triggering RLS (eg, [43–45]) and may occur in younger and older patients. Neuropathies and radiculopathies, disorders normally of older age, have been reported to be associated with RLS and have generally been acknowledged as possible underlying causes of RLS [25,46,47], though supporting data for this presumption is limited [48]. Rheumatoid arthritis has been reported to be associated with a 25% incidence of RLS [49]. Further conditions, possibly causally related to RLS, include chronic obstructive pulmonary disease, asthma [48], fibromyalgia [50], and diabetes mellitus [41].

RLS can also occur in several neurodegenerative disorders, such as in Parkinson's disease [51–54], multiple system atrophy [51] or spinocerebellar ataxia [55], and disorders usually occurring in middle-aged or elderly patients. RLS is also more frequent in patients with multiple sclerosis [56], and leg restlessness appears to be one of the most common reasons for sleep disturbances in cancer patients [57,58]. In addition, the prevalence of mental disorders, most often depression and anxiety disorders, has been found to be increased by 1.5 to 2 times in RLS, compared with the non-RLS affected population [48,59,60]. RLS may also occur or worsen because of the effect of some pharmacologic agents. A summary of case reports and case series reporting on medication-triggered or worsened RLS is presented in Table 1.

Treatment of restless legs syndrome in the elderly

The most commonly prescribed drugs for RLS with dosing and side effects are presented in Table 2. No studies investigated treatment effect specifically in the elderly. The treatment of RLS is a symptomatic one, as the pathophysiology of RLS is not yet known. According to the timely occurrence of symptoms, RLS medications are usually taken at bedtime.

The pathophysiology of RLS has been related to the dopaminergic system [61–63]. Indeed, several studies have shown significant improvement of RLS in clinical studies using dopaminergic agents, and levodopa and

Table 1
Case reports and case series reporting on medication triggered or worsened RLS

Substance	Publication*
Cimetidine	O'Sullivan and Greenberg, 1993
Citalopram	Nader, et al, 2007
Clozapine	Duggal and Mendhekar, 2007
Flunarizine	Micheli, et al, 1989
Fluoxetine	Bakshi, 1996
Haloperidol	Horiguchi, et al, 1999
Interferon-alpha	LaRochelle and Karp, 2004
Caffeine	Lutz, 1978
Lithium	Heiman and Christie, 1986; Terao, et al, 1991
L-thyroxine	Tan, et al, 2004
Methsuximide and Phenytoin	Drake, 1988
Mianserin	Paik, et al, 1989; Markkula and Lauerma, 1997
Mirtazapine	Bonin, et al, 2000; Bahk, et al, 2002; Teive, et al, 2002; Agargun, et al, 2002
Olanzapine	Kraus, et al, 1999
Paroxetine	Sanz-Fuentenebro, et al, 1996
Quetiapine	Pinninti, et al, 2005
Risperidone	Wetter, et al, 2002
Saccharine	De Groot, 2006
Sertraline	Hargrave and Beckley, 1998

* *Adapted from* Trenkwalder C, Benes H, Hornyak M, et al. Restless legs syndrom und periodic limb movement disorder. In: Diener CH, editor. Leitlinien für Diagnostik und Therapie in der Neurologie, 4th edition. Stuttgart: Thieme; in press.

dopamine agonists are considered to be the treatment of choice in RLS [64–68]. The dopamine precursor levodopa in combination with a dopa-decarboxylase inhibitor, is an effective therapeutic agent with high tolerability and without serious side effects, also in patients with concomitant

Table 2
Dopaminergic medications for the treatment of RLS

Medication	Daily dose rate	Side effects
Levodopa + dopa-decarboxylase inhibitor	100 mg–400 mg + 25 mg–100 mg	Diarrhea, nausea, dyspepsia, reduced general drive, muscle weakness, somnolence, headache
Pramipexole	0.088 mg–0.54 mg	Nausea, dizziness, fatigue, somnolence, headache, orthostatic hypotension
Ropinirole	0.25 mg–4 mg	Nausea, dizziness, fatigue, somnolence, headache, orthostatic hypotension
Rotigotine (transdermal patches)	0.5 mg–4.5 mg	Nausea, dizziness, fatigue, skin reactions at the patch site, orthostatic hypotension
Cabergoline	0.5 mg–2.0 mg	Nausea, dizziness, fatigue, somnolence, headache, orthostatic hypotension, cardiac valvular disease
Pergolide	0.25 mg–0.75 mg (mean 0.51 mg)	Nausea, dizziness, fatigue, somnolence, headache, orthostatic hypotension, cardiac valvular disease

medical disorders. It has been shown that levodopa improves RLS symptoms, quality of sleep, and quality of life [69]. Furthermore, the benefit of dopaminergic agonists in RLS has been proven in several studies (for a recent review, see Ref. [68]). Their use, however, may be limited in the elderly because of possible interactions with multiple other medications and of side effects, such as orthostatic hypotension, nausea, or dizziness.

Pramipexole [70–72] and ropinirole [73–75] are the most extensively studied drugs for RLS, and the only dopamine agonists that are approved by the Food and Drug Administration (FDA) for the treatment of RLS. Unfortunately, most studies on these drugs have been conducted in nonelderly populations. Whether the results can be extrapolated to older adults is uncertain. Several large, randomized controlled trials have been published, however the mean age of study subjects was 50 to 60 years. These studies do indicate significant benefits, as measured by International Restless Legs Syndrome (IRLS), Clinical Global Impression-Improvement (CGI-I), and Quality of Life scales.

A 12-week randomized controlled study of ropinirole versus placebo was recently published [74]. The mean subject age was 54 to 56 years. In this study of 267 subjects, the treatment group had a reduction in IRLS score (range 0–40) at week one, by a clinically significant 8.4 points from a baseline of 24. This improvement continued and increased in magnitude through the first 8 weeks of treatment. The CGI-I score (1, very much improved to 7, very much worse) also improved "much" or "very much" in 59.5% of the subjects in the treatment group, versus 39.6% of the placebo subjects (odds ratio 2.3; 95% confidence interval, 1.4–3.8, $P = 0.001$).

In the nearly identical study of 284 subjects published the same year by Trenkwalder and colleagues [73], IRLS score improved by 11.0 versus 8.0 points over 12 weeks ($P < 0.01$). The percent with "much" or "very much" improved CGI-I score was 53.4%, versus 40.9% in the placebo group ($P < 0.05$). In a smaller long-term efficacy study, 202 subjects received ropinirole for 24 weeks and treatment or placebo for a further 12 weeks [76]. The primary outcome was percentage with symptom relapse at 36 weeks. Significantly fewer patients relapsed on ropinirole than on placebo (32.6% versus 57.8%, $P < 0.05$).

Pramipexole has demonstrated symptomatic benefit similar to ropinirole. In a 12-week study by Winkelman and colleagues [70], 344 subjects (mean age 51.4) were randomized to three doses of pramipexole versus placebo. At study completion, mean improvement in IRLS score was 4.3 points better in the treated groups as compared with placebo ($P < 0.01$). There were no IRLS score differences between pramipexole dosing groups. The percentage of subjects "much" or "very much" better on CGI-I score was 72.0%, versus 51.2% in the placebo group ($P < 0.01$). In a smaller study, 109 subjects were followed for 3 weeks on pramipaxole versus placebo. Treated subjects had significantly improved IRLS scores and CGI-I scores when compared with placebo [71].

While nonergot derivates (pramipexol, ropinirole) have emerged as the first-line option when dopamine agonists are indicated, the ergot derivates (eg, cabergoline, pergolide) are more infrequently used because of an increased risk of valvular heart disease [77]. On March 29, 2007, the FDA announced a recall of pergolide from the United States market because of the risk of serious valvular heart disease. Recent studies have linked pergolide with increased chance of regurgitation of the mitral, tricuspid, and aortic valves.

Both cabergoline [78,79] and pergolide [80] are effective in improving RLS symptoms significantly and can be used as second-line treatment when nonergot derivates are not sufficient. In a 2004 study of pergolide, 100 subjects (mean age 56.2) entered a 6-week double-blind placebo-controlled phase followed by a 10.5-month open label pergolide phase for prior nonresponders [80]. At 6 weeks, the pergolide group demonstrated improved IRLS and CGI-I scores ($P < 0.001$). During phase 2, treated subjects maintained symptom improvement, and previous nonresponders switching to pergolide exhibited improvement in the periodic limb movement index.

Two studies of cabergoline in RLS demonstrate both subjective and objective improvement in RLS symptoms. In one study, 85 subjects (mean age 56) were randomized to one of three treatment doses of cabergoline and placebo for 5 weeks of treatment, followed by a 42-week open label phase. Treated subjects showed improvement in RLS-6 scales and IRLS score, compared with placebo over the initial 5 weeks. At 1 year, cabergoline subjects had improved sleep quality compared with baseline values [78]. In another 5-week protocol, subjects randomized to cabergoline had fewer periodic leg movements ($P = 0.001$), better sleep efficiency ($P = 0.044$), and longer total sleep time ($P = 0.044$) than placebo [79].

An alternate route is available for treating RLS via transdermal application of dopamine agonists. This route of administration ensures a constant rate of drug delivery, more steady serum concentration, and reduction in daytime breakthrough symptoms. This treatment option may be especially useful in patients experiencing severe RLS with symptoms over most of the day. Transdermal formulations include the dopamine agonists lisuride and rotigotine.

Lisuride was studied in nine subjects (mean age 58) for 1 week after a 2-week open-label run-in phase. IRLS and CGI-I scales improved in the 1 week treated group compared with placebo [81]. Rotigotine was studied in 63 subjects for 1 week at three different treatment doses. At the highest dose of 4.5 mg, rotigotine reduced IRLS score by 15.7 points, versus 8 points in the placebo group ($P < 0.01$). According to the RLS-6 scales, daytime symptoms were improved with all rotigotine doses [82].

Up to now there have been no published comparative studies of dopamine agonists and no long-term studies exceeding a 1-year treatment period. The most clinically relevant problem with levodopa and dopamine agonists in treating RLS is the development of augmentation phenomena [4,83]. The main characteristic of augmentation is the medication use-related increase of symptoms, which typically occurs after an initial improvement [4]. In patients with augmentation, elevating the dosage of the dopaminergic substance associated with the augmentation usually leads to a transient relief of symptoms, sometimes lasting only for a few weeks. Augmentation is probably a dopaminergic treatment-related phenomenon, although a recent case report described a similar side effect during opiate therapy [84]. The occurrence of augmentation usually demands a switch to another drug.

Opioids seem to have a long-term efficacy in the treatment of RLS and are well tolerated in the elderly [67]; however, the number of clinical studies with opioids is limited. Oxycodone is the best studied opioid for improving RLS symptoms [68]. Clinical or polysomnographic monitoring for the development of sleep apnea is recommended in patients on long-term opioid therapy [67]. Patients with painful paresthesias may respond positively to anticonvulsants, such as gabapentine [85,86]. Benzodiazepines and benzodiazepine-like hypnotics, such as zopiclone or zolpidem, may also improve sleep in RLS patients, mainly in those with less severe symptoms. However, hypnotics need special attention when prescribed in the elderly [65]. There is some evidence that iron supplementation with intravenous iron dextran is effective in low-ferritin patients and in patients with RLS secondary to uraemia [87,88]. Magnesium was found effective to decrease PLMS in a pilot study investigating RLS patients and insomniacs with elevated PLMS [89].

Summary

Restless legs syndrome is a clinical diagnosis with an estimated 9% to 20% prevalence in the elderly. A detailed history of the patient, and if necessary of the caregivers, is important in the diagnosis. RLS should be considered in the differential diagnosis of any older patient with sleep disturbances or paresthesias of the limbs. The high association of RLS with several disorders has to be born in mind. Some pharmacologic agents could also trigger or exacerbate RLS. Dopaminergic drugs are the first-line treatment option in RLS. The most clinically relevant problem with dopaminergic drugs in treating RLS is the development of augmentation, a medication use-related increase of symptoms, which usually occurs after an initial improvement and demands a switch of medication.

References

[1] Hening W, Walters AS, Allen RP, et al. Impact, diagnosis and treatment of restless legs syndrome (RLS) in a primary care population: the REST (RLS epidemiology, symptoms, and treatment) primary care study. Sleep Med 2004;5(3):237–46.

[2] McCrink L, Allen RP, Wolowacz S, et al. Predictors of health-related quality of life in sufferers with restless legs syndrome: a multi-national study. Sleep Med 2007;8(1):73–83.

[3] Walters AS. The International Restless Legs Syndrome Study Group. Toward a better definition of the Restless Legs Syndrome. Mov Disord 1995;10(5):634–42.

[4] Allen RP, Picchietti D, Hening WA, et al. Restless legs syndrome: diagnostic criteria, special considerations and epidemiology. A report from the restless legs syndrome diagnosis and epidemiology workshop at the National Institute of Health. Sleep Med 2003;4(2): 101–19.

[5] Hornyak M, Feige B, Voderholzer U, et al. Polysomnography findings in patients with restless legs syndrome and in healthy controls: a comparative observational study. Sleep 2007; 30(7):861–5.

[6] Montplaisir J, Boucher S, Poirier G, et al. Clinical, polysomnographic, and genetic characteristics of restless legs syndrome: a study of 133 patients diagnosed with new standard criteria. Mov Disord 1997;12(1):61–5.

[7] Bonnet M, Carley D, Carskadon M, et al. Atlas Task Force of the American Sleep Disorders Association. Recording and scoring leg movements. Sleep 1993;16(8):748–59.

[8] Zucconi M, Ferri R, Allen R, et al. International Restless Legs Syndrome Study Group (IRLSSG). The official World Association of Sleep Medicine (WASM) standards for recording and scoring periodic leg movements in sleep (PLMS) and wakefulness (PLMW) developed in collaboration with a task force from the International Restless Legs Syndrome Study Group (IRLSSG). Sleep Med 2006;7(2):175–83.

[9] de Weerd AW, Rijsman RM, Brinkley A. Activity patterns of leg muscles in periodic limb movement disorder. J Neurol Neurosurg Psychiatry 2004;75(2):317–9.

[10] Coleman RM. Periodic movements in sleep (nocturnal myoclonus) and restless legs syndrome. In: Guilleminault C, editor. Sleep and waking disorders: indications and techniques. Menlo Park (CA): Addison-Wesley Publishing Company; 1982. p. 265–95.

[11] Hornyak M, Feige B, Riemann D, et al. Periodic leg movements in sleep and periodic limb movement disorder: prevalence, clinical significance and treatment. Sleep Med Rev 2006; 10(3):169–77.

[12] Montplaisir J, Godbout R. Nocturnal sleep of narcoleptic patients. Sleep 1986;9(1 Pt 2): 159–61.

[13] Ferri R, Zucconi M, Manconi M, et al. Different periodicity and time structure of leg movements during sleep in narcolepsy/cataplexy and restless legs syndrome. Sleep 2006;29(12): 1587–94.

[14] Fry JM, DiPhilippo MA, Pressmann MR. Periodic leg movements in sleep following treatment of obstructive sleep apnea with nasal continuous positive airway pressure. Chest 1989; 96(1):89–91.

[15] Fantini ML, Michaud M, Gosselin N, et al. Periodic leg movements in REM sleep behavior disorder and related autonomic and EEG activation. Neurology 2002;59(12):1889–94.

[16] Carrier J, Frenette S, Montplaisir J, et al. Effects of periodic leg movements during sleep in middle-aged subjects without sleep complaints. Mov Disord 2005;20(9):1127–32.

[17] Pearson VE, Allen RP, Dean T, et al. Cognitive deficits associated with restless legs syndrome (RLS). Sleep Med 2006;7(1):25–30.

[18] Walters AS, Hening W, Rubinstein M, et al. A clinical and polysomnographic comparison of neuroleptic-induced akathisia and the idiopathic restless legs syndrome. Sleep 1991;14(4): 339–45.

[19] Picchietti DL, Walters AS. Moderate to severe periodic limb movement disorder in childhood and adolescence. Sleep 1999;22(3):297–300.

[20] Walters AS, Hickey K, Maltzman J, et al. A questionnaire study of 138 patients with restless legs syndrome: the "night walkers" survey. Neurology 1996;46(1):92–5.

[21] Allen RP, Earley CJ. Defining the phenotype of the restless legs syndrome (RLS) using age-of-symptom-onset. Sleep Med 2000;1(1):11–9.

[22] Winkelmann J, Muller-Myhsok B, Wittchen HU, et al. Complex segregation analysis of restless legs syndrome provides evidence for an autosomal dominant mode of inheritance in early age at onset families. Ann Neurol 2002;52(3):297–302.

[23] Hanson M, Honour M, Singleton A, et al. Analysis of familial and sporadic restless legs syndrome in age of onset, gender, and severity features. J Neurol 2004;251(11):1398–401.

[24] Kotagal S, Silber MH. Childhood-onset restless legs syndrome. Ann Neurol 2004;56(6): 803–7.

[25] Polydefkis M, Allen RP, Hauer P, et al. Subclinical sensory neuropathy in late-onset restless legs syndrome. Neurology 2000;55(8):1115–21.

[26] Ondo WG, Vuong KD, Wang Q. Restless legs syndrome in monozygotic twins: clinical correlates. Neurology 2000;55(9):1404–6.

[27] Winkelmann J, Wetter TC, Collado-Seidel V, et al. Clinical characteristics and frequency of the hereditary restless legs syndrome in a population of 300 patients. Sleep 2000;23(5): 597–602.

[28] Earley CJ, Connor JR, Beard JL, et al. Ferritin levels in the cerebrospinal fluid and restless legs syndrome: effects of different clinical phenotypes. Sleep 2005;28(9):1069–75.

[29] Earley CJ, Barker PB, Horska A, et al. MRI-determined regional brain iron concentrations in early- and late-onset restless legs syndrome. Sleep Med 2006;7(5):458–61.

[30] Berger K, von Eckardstein A, Trenkwalder C, et al. Iron metabolism and the risk of restless legs syndrome in an elderly general population—The MEMO study. J Neurol 2002;249(9): 1195–9.

[31] O'Keeffe ST. Secondary causes of restless legs syndrome in older people. Age Ageing 2005; 34(4):349–52.

[32] Bassetti CL, Mauerhofer D, Gugger M, et al. Restless legs syndrome: a clinical study of 55 patients. Eur Neurol 2001;45(2):67–74.

[33] Lavigne GJ, Montplaisir JY. Restless legs syndrome and sleep bruxism: prevalence and association among Canadians. Sleep 1994;17(8):739–43.

[34] Phillips B, Young T, Finn L, et al. Epidemiology of restless legs symptoms in adults. Arch Intern Med 2000;160(14):2137–41.

[35] Ulfberg J, Nyström B, Carter N, et al. Prevalence of restless legs syndrome among men aged 18 to 64 years: an association with somatic disease and neuropsychiatric symptoms. Mov Disord 2001;16(6):1159–63.

[36] Ohayon MM, Roth T. Prevalence of restless legs syndrome and periodic limb movement disorder in the general population. J Psychosom Res 2002;53(1):547–54.

[37] Tison F, Crochard A, Leger D, et al. Epidemiology of restless legs syndrome in French adults: a nationwide survey: the INSTANT Study. Neurology 2005;65(2):239–46.

[38] Bjorvatn B, Leissner L, Ulfberg J, et al. Prevalence, severity and risk factors of restless legs syndrome in the general adult population in two Scandinavian countries. Sleep Med 2005; 6(4):307–12.

[39] Winkelman JW, Finn L, Young T. Prevalence and correlates of restless legs syndrome symptoms in the Wisconsin Sleep Cohort. Sleep Med 2006;7(7):545–52.

[40] Rothdach AJ, Trenkwalder C, Haberstock J, et al. Prevalence and risk factors of RLS in an elderly population. The MEMO study. Neurology 2000;54(5):1064–8.

[41] Berger K, Luedemann J, Trenkwalder C, et al. Sex and the risk of restless legs syndrome in the general population. Arch Intern Med 2004;164(2):196–202.

[42] Högl B, Kiechl S, Willeit J, et al. Restless legs syndrome: a community-based study of prevalence, severity, and risk factors. Neurology 2005;64(11):1920–4.

[43] Ekbom KA. Restless legs syndrome. Neurology 1960;10:868–73.

[44] Roger SD, Harris DCH, Stewart JH. Possible relation between restless legs and anemia in renal dialysis patients. Lancet 1991;337(8756):1551.

[45] Rijsman RM, de Weerd AW, Stam CJ, et al. Periodic limb movement disorder and restless legs syndrome in dialysis patients. Nephrology 2004;9(6):353–61.

[46] Iannaccone S, Zucconi M, Marchettini P, et al. Evidence of peripheral axonal neuropathy in primary restless legs syndrome. Mov Disord 1995;10(1):2–9.

[47] Gemignani F, Brindani F, Negrotti A, et al. Restless legs syndrome and polyneuropathy. Mov Disord 2006;21(8):1254–7.

[48] Banno K, Delaive K, Walld R, et al. Restless legs syndrome in 218 patients: associated disorders. Sleep Med 2000;1(3):221–9.

[49] Salih AM, Gray RE, Mills KR, et al. A clinical, serological and neurophysiological study of restless legs syndrome in rheumatoid arthritis. Br J Rheumatol 1994;33(1):60–3.

[50] Yunus M, Aldag J. Restless legs syndrome and leg cramps in fibromyalgia syndrome—a controlled study. BMJ 1996;312(7042):339–40.

[51] Wetter TC, Collado-Seidel V, Pollmacher T, et al. Sleep and periodic leg movement patterns in drug-free patients with Parkinson's disease and multiple system atrophy. Sleep 2000;23(3): 361–7.

[52] Tan EK, Lum SY, Wong MC. Restless legs syndrome in Parkinson's disease. J Neurol Sci 2002;196(1–2):33–6.

[53] Nomura T, Inoue Y, Nakashima K. Clinical characteristics of Restless legs syndrome in patients with Parkinson's disease. J Neurol Sci 2006;250(1–2):39–44.

[54] Wszolek ZK, Brown LA. Prevalence and clinical characteristics of restless legs syndrome in Japanese patients with Parkinson's disease. Mov Disord 2007;22(2):284.

[55] Abele M, Burk K, Laccone F, et al. Restless legs syndrome in spinocerebellar ataxia types 1, 2, and 3. J Neurol 2001;248(4):311–4.

[56] Auger C, Montplaisir J, Duquette P. Increased frequency of restless legs syndrome in a French-Canadian population with multiple sclerosis. Neurology 2005;65(10):1652–3.

[57] Silberfarb PM, Hauri PJ, Oxmann TE, et al. Assessment of sleep in patients with lung cancer and breast cancer. J Clin Oncol 1993;11(5):997–1004.

[58] Davidson JR, MacLean AW, Brundage MD, et al. Sleep disturbance in cancer patients. Soc Sci Med 2002;54(9):1309–21.

[59] Winkelmann J, Prager M, Lieb R, et al. "Anxietas tibiarum". Depression and anxiety disorders in patients with restless legs syndrome. J Neurol 2005;252(1):67–71.

[60] Phillips B, Hening W, Britz P, et al. Prevalence and correlates of restless legs syndrome: results from the 2005 National Sleep Foundation Poll. Chest 2006;129(1):76–80.

[61] Walters AS, Hening WA. Review of the clinical presentation and the neuropharmacology of the restless legs syndrome. Clin Neuropharmacol 1987;10(3):225–37.

[62] Montplaisir J, Lorrain D, Godbout R. Restless legs syndrome and periodic leg movements in sleep: the primary role of dopaminergic mechanism. Eur Neurol 1991;31(1):41–3.

[63] Trenkwalder C, Paulus W. Why do restless legs occur at rest?–pathophysiology of neuronal structures in RLS. Neurophysiology of RLS (part 2). Clin Neurophysiol 2004;115(9): 1975–88.

[64] Chesson AL Jr, Wise M, Davila D, et al. Practice parameters for the treatment of restless legs syndrome and periodic limb movement disorder. An American Academy of Sleep Medicine Report. Standards of Practice Committee of the American Academy of Sleep Medicine. Sleep 1999;22(7):961–8.

[65] Hening W, Allen R, Earley C, et al. The treatment of restless legs syndrome and periodic limb movement disorder—an American Academy of Sleep Medicine Review. Sleep 1999;22(7): 970–98.

[66] Stiasny K, Oertel WH, Trenkwalder C. Clinical symptomatology and treatment of restless legs syndrome and periodic limb movement disorder. Sleep Med Rev 2002;6(4):253–65.

[67] Walters AS, Winkelmann J, Trenkwalder C, et al. Long-term follow-up on restless legs syndrome patients treated with opioids. Mov Disord 2001;16(6):1105–9.

[68] Vignatelli L, Billiard M, Clarenbach P, et al. EFNS guidelines on management of restless legs syndrome and periodic limb movement disorder in sleep. Eur J Neurol 2006;13(10): 1049–65.

[69] Benes H, Kurella B, Kummer J, et al. Rapid onset of action of levodopa in restless legs syndrome: a double-blind, randomized, multicenter, crossover trial. Sleep 1999;22(8): 1073–81.

[70] Winkelman JW, Sethi D, Kushida CA, et al. Efficacy and safety of pramipexole in restless legs syndrome. Neurology 2006;67(6):1034–9.

[71] Partinen M, Hirvonen K, Jama L, et al. Efficacy and safety of pramipexole in idiopathic restless legs syndrome: a polysomnographic dose-finding study–the PRELUDE study. Sleep Med 2006;7(5):407–17.

[72] Oertel WH, Stiasny-Kolster K, Bergtholdt B, et al. Efficacy of pramipexole in restless legs syndrome: a six-week, multicenter, randomized, double-blind study (effect-RLS study). Mov Disord 2007;22(2):213–9.

[73] Trenkwalder C, Garcia-Borreguero D, Montagna P, et al. Ropinirole in the treatment of restless legs syndrome: results from the TREAT RLS 1 study, a 12 week, randomised, placebo controlled study in 10 European countries. J Neurol Neurosurg Psychiatry 2004; 75(1):92–7.

[74] Walters AS, Ondo WG, Dreykluft T, et al. Ropinirole is effective in the treatment of restless legs syndrome. TREAT RLS 2: a 12-week, double-blind, randomized, parallel-group, placebo-controlled study. Mov Disord 2004;19(12):1414–23.

[75] Bogan RK, Fry JM, Schmidt MH, et al. Ropinirole in the treatment of patients with restless legs syndrome: a US-based randomized, double-blind, placebo-controlled clinical trial. Mayo Clin Proc 2006;81(1):17–27.

[76] Montplaisir J, Karrasch J, Haan J, et al. Ropinirole is effective in the long-term management of restless legs syndrome: a randomized controlled trial. Mov Disord 2006;21(10):1627–35.

[77] Zanettini R, Antonini A, Gatto G, et al. Valvular heart disease and the use of dopamine agonists for Parkinson's disease. N Engl J Med 2007;356(1):39–46.

[78] Stiasny-Kolster K, Benes H, Peglau I, et al. Effective cabergoline treatment in idiopathic restless legs syndrome. Neurology 2004;63(12):2272–9.

[79] Oertel WH, Benes H, Bodenschatz R, et al. Efficacy of cabergoline in restless legs syndrome: a placebo-controlled study with polysomnography (CATOR). Neurology 2006;67(6): 1040–6.

[80] Trenkwalder C, Hundemer HP, Lledo A, et al. Efficacy of pergolide in treatment of restless legs syndrome: the PEARLS Study. Neurology 2004;62(8):1391–7.

[81] Benes H. Transdermal lisuride: short-term efficacy and tolerability study in patients with severe restless legs syndrome. Sleep Med 2006;7(1):31–5.

[82] Stiasny-Kolster K, Kohnen R, Schollmayer E, et al. Patch application of the dopamine agonist rotigotine to patients with moderate to advanced stages of restless legs syndrome. Mov Disord 2004;19(12):1432–8.

[83] Paulus W, Trenkwalder C. Less is more: pathophysiology of dopaminergic-therapy-related augmentation in restless legs syndrome. Lancet Neurology 2006;5(10):878–86.

[84] Vetrugno R, La Morgia C, D'Angelo R, et al. Augmentation of restless legs syndrome with long-term tramadol treatment. Mov Disord 2007;22(3):424–7.

[85] Happe S, Klosch G, Saletu B, et al. Treatment of idiopathic restless legs syndrome (RLS) with gabapentin. Neurology 2001;57(9):1717–9.

[86] Garcia-Borreguero D, Larrosa O, de la Llave Y, et al. Treatment of restless legs syndrome with gabapentin: a double-blind, cross-over study. Neurology 2002;59(10):1573–9.

[87] Earley CJ, Heckler D, Allen RP. The treatment of restless legs syndrome with intravenous iron dextran. Sleep Med 2004;5(3):231–5.

[88] Sloand JA, Shelly MA, Feigin A, et al. A double-blind, placebo-controlled trial of intravenous iron dextran therapy in patients with ESRD and restless legs syndrome. Am J Kidney Dis 2004;43(4):663–70.

[89] Hornyak M, Voderholzer U, Hohagen F, et al. Magnesium therapy for periodic leg movements-related insomnia and restless legs syndrome: an open pilot study. Sleep 1998;21(5): 501–5.

ELSEVIER
SAUNDERS

Clin Geriatr Med 24 (2008) 181–184

CLINICS IN
GERIATRIC
MEDICINE

Index

Note: Page numbers of article titles are in **boldface** type.

0749-0690/08/$ - see front matter © 2008 Elsevier Inc. All rights reserved.
doi:10.1016/S0749-0690(07)00101-2

geriatric.theclinics.com

Moving?

Make sure your subscription moves with you!

To notify us of your new address, find your **Clinics Account Number** (located on your mailing label above your name), and contact customer service at:

E-mail: elspcs@elsevier.com

800-654-2452 (subscribers in the U.S. & Canada)
314-453-7041 (subscribers outside of the U.S. & Canada)

Fax number: 314-523-5170

Elsevier Periodicals Customer Service
11830 Westline Industrial Drive
St. Louis, MO 63146

*To ensure uninterrupted delivery of your subscription, please notify us at least 4 weeks in advance of move.

Printed and bound by CPI Group (UK) Ltd, Croydon, CR0 4YY

03/10/2024

01040462-0016